Anxious Geographies

Anxious Geographies offers a unique perspective on social anxiety, framing it as both a social and spatial phenomenon. Through a meticulous exploration using online questionnaires and interviews, the book provides a crucial examination of the intricacies of anxious lives.

This book presents a critical intervention in the experience of mental health in 21st-century society and provides a compelling geographical account of the underpinnings of the anxious experience. The book pivots on the in-depth perspectives of people with social anxiety, diagnosed or "sub-clinical", but with an academic commentary that relates their experience to the medicalisation of a disrupted relational life, offering lessons for all of us in modern societies. Each chapter considers a unique aspect of social anxiety accounting for the social, spatial, temporal, relational and embodied dynamics, a geographical approach that enriches our understanding of the contexts and conditions that exacerbate and sustain anxious distress. The phenomenological descriptions herein, capture how social anxiety can profoundly alter a person's coherent, habitual and embodied sense of being in and navigating through their social and spatial worlds. Through the experiential accounts of anxious distress and by considering the social contexts in which they emerge, this book provides readers with crucial insights into the hidden lives of those living with social anxiety.

This book will be of appeal to academics, researchers and postgraduate students in the fields of human geography and across the social sciences and humanities. It will also provide useful insights for academics and health professionals in social psychiatry, social psychology, counselling studies and therapeutic practice.

Louise E. Boyle is an honorary research fellow in the School of Geographical and Earth Sciences at the University of Glasgow, Scotland. She has published in Social Science and Medicine and co-edited the forthcoming Routledge Handbook on Spaces of Mental Health and Well-Being (2024).

Geographies of Health

Edited by Allison Williams, *Associate Professor, School of Geography and Earth Sciences, McMaster University, Canada*, and **Susan Elliott**, *Professor, Department of Geography and Environmental Management and School of Public Health and Health Systems, University of Waterloo, Canada*

There is growing interest in the geographies of health and a continued interest in what has more traditionally been labelled medical geography. The traditional focus of "medical geography" on areas such as disease ecology, health service provision and disease mapping (all of which continue to reflect a mainly quantitative approach to inquiry) has evolved to a focus on a broader, theoretically informed epistemology of health geographies in an expanded international reach. As a result, we now find this subdiscipline characterised by a strongly theoretically informed research agenda, embracing a range of methods (quantitative, qualitative and the integration of the two) of inquiry concerned with questions of: risk; representation and meaning; inequality and power; culture and difference, among others. Health mapping and modelling have simultaneously been strengthened by the technical advances made in multilevel modelling, advanced spatial analytic methods and GIS, while further engaging in questions related to health inequalities, population health and environmental degradation.

This series publishes superior-quality research monographs and edited collections representing contemporary applications in the field; this encompasses original research as well as advances in methods, techniques and theories. The *Geographies of Health* series will capture the interest of a broad body of scholars, within the social sciences, the health sciences and beyond.

Blue Space, Health and Wellbeing
Hydrophilia Unbounded
Edited by Ronan Foley, Robin Kearns, Thomas Kistemann and Ben Wheeler

Cultivated Therapeutic Landscapes
Gardening for Prevention, Restoration and Equity
Edited by Pauline Marsh and Allison Williams

Equity in Global Health Research
Edited by Elijah Bisung and Katrina Plamondon

Anxious Geographies
Worlds of Social Anxiety
Louise E. Boyle

For a full list of titles in this series, please visit https://www.routledge.com/Geographies-of-Health-Series/book-series/GHS

Anxious Geographies

Worlds of Social Anxiety

Louise E. Boyle

Routledge
Taylor & Francis Group

LONDON AND NEW YORK

First published 2024
by Routledge
4 Park Square, Milton Park, Abingdon, Oxon OX14 4RN

and by Routledge
605 Third Avenue, New York, NY 10158

Routledge is an imprint of the Taylor & Francis Group, an informa business

British Library Cataloguing-in-Publication Data
A catalogue record for this book is available from the British Library

Library of Congress Cataloging-in-Publication Data
Names: Boyle, Louise E., author.
Title: Anxious geographies : worlds of social anxiety / Louise E. Boyle.
Description: Abingdon, Oxon ; New York, NY : Routledge, 2024. |
Series:Geographies of health series | Includes bibliographical references and index.
Identifiers: LCCN 2023055467 (print) | LCCN 2023055468 (ebook) |
ISBN 9781032074313 (hardback) | ISBN 9781032074368 (paperback) |
ISBN 9781003206880 (ebook)
Subjects: LCSH: Social phobia. | Social phobia--Patients. | Social
phobia--Patients--Social networks. | Social phobia--Patients--Social
conditions. | Social psychiatry. | Boyle, Louise E.--Mental health.
Classification: LCC RC552.S62 B695 2024 (print) | LCC RC552.S62
(ebook) | DDC 616.85/225--dc23/eng/20240123
LC record available at https://lccn.loc.gov/2023055467
LC ebook record available at https://lccn.loc.gov/2023055468

ISBN: 978-1-032-07431-3 (hbk)
ISBN: 978-1-032-07436-8 (pbk)
ISBN: 978-1-003-20688-0 (ebk)

DOI: 10.4324/9781003206880

Typeset in Times New Roman
by SPi Technologies India Pvt Ltd (Straive)

Contents

Preface

In May 2021, as I began work on this book, the world number two tennis champion Naomi Osaka announced that she would not be participating in press conferences and media interviews for the remainder of the French Open, normally a contractual requirement of competing in an international tennis tournament, citing her mental health, specifically the exacerbating effects of these activities on her social anxiety. She noted elsewhere that "she does not court the spotlight" because the intensity of the "traditional format of the press conference", specifically the "subject vs. object" approach, "comes at a cost of great anxiety" (Osaka, 2021). The challenges she faced were recognisable to anyone with social anxiety. Being the subject of others' scrutiny, experiencing the immense pressure of performing, feeling exposed and vulnerable to others' judgements are no doubt amplified by being under the glare of the world's press. This is especially true in environments that, as the fallout from her announcement demonstrated, are at best uncomfortable with, or at worst, hostile to expressions or discussions of mental health. It was the first time, as far as I could remember, that a public figure and notable sportsperson had spoken openly and candidly about social anxiety and the impact it was having on her ability to manage the roles and responsibilities that many would consider to be part of everyday life. I was cautiously optimistic, conscious of the very real stigma surrounding social anxiety, that this could be an opportunity to combat mischaracterisations and raise public awareness of the many unseen challenges people face navigating daily life. Yet, while support arrived from peers and from pockets of the media, as well as from the general public, any hope that this could be a turning point for understanding of social anxiety was short-lived. In a subsequent statement, Roland Garros (the tournament organiser) reprimanded Osaka in a public statement, warning her:

> that should she continue to ignore her media obligations during the tournament, she would be exposing herself to possible further Code of Conduct infringement consequences [...] As might be expected, repeated violations attract tougher sanctions including default from the tournament and the trigger of a major offence investigation that could lead to more substantial fines and future Grand Slam suspensions.
>
> (2021)

As she "chose not to honour her contractual obligations", she was issued with a \$15,000 fine. In light of this, she made the subsequent decision to withdraw from the tournament entirely. In a public statement made via her Twitter account, she said:

> I think now the best thing [...] is that I withdraw so that everyone can get back to focusing on the tennis [...] I never wanted to be a distraction [...] Anyone that knows me knows I'm introverted, and anyone that has seen me at tournaments will notice that I'm often wearing headphones as that helps dull my social anxiety [...] I am not a natural public speaker and get huge waves of anxiety before I speak to the world's media. I get really nervous and find it stressful to always try to engage and give you the best answers I can. So here in Paris I was already feeling vulnerable and anxious so I thought it was better to exercise self-care and skip the press conferences. I announced it pre-emptively because I do feel like the rules are quite outdated in parts and I wanted to highlight that.
>
> (Osaka [@naomiosaka] 2021)

While Osaka's anxiety surrounding press conferences and public speaking coupled with her ultimate decision to withdraw may seem extreme and unnecessary, they are entirely relatable to someone living with social anxiety. Unfortunately, what was even more relatable was the response from Roland Garros who, while noting in the same statement that players' mental health is of the "utmost importance", managed further to isolate and ultimately exclude Osaka from the tournament, threatening her with further sanctions, investigations, fines and suspensions. These are repercussions, that in any setting, would have a devastating impact not only on a person's health and wellbeing, but their very sense of self. At a later press conference, she commented that she had spent the following weeks "holed up in my house [...] embarrassed to go out, because I didn't know if people were looking at me in a different way" (Osaka cited in Daugherty, 2021). Social anxiety often leaves a person feeling vulnerable, hopelessly exposed to the scrutiny of others, and critics seem unable to see the consequences for the person concerned about their anxiety playing out on the world stage. It would be fair to say that Osaka already felt exposed prior to her announcement, and so, the decision to discuss her anxiety publicly, let alone to announce to the world that she was taking a temporary break from her media obligations to manage it better, is absolutely not one that would have been taken lightly.

While the coverage on social media was generally positive, in terms of affirming others experiences, critiquing existing structures that are detrimental to mental health and destigmatising through visibility, there was an all too familiar dismissal of mental health – and specifically a lack of understanding of social anxiety – permeating much of the surrounding discourse (Kumble, Diddi and Bien-Aimé, 2022). Osaka is also a young Haitian-American and Japanese female athlete and her decision, and the subsequent backlash, also sparked intense discussion about race, gender, health and power relations in sport and beyond (Tuakli-Wosornu and Darling-Hammond, 2022). Osaka suffered repeated dismissal of her mental health and further public humiliation at the hands of individuals and organisations, which put her wellbeing at further risk. The French Tennis Federation (FTF) succeeded not only in trivialising social anxiety as a personal choice but further admonished her as someone shirking her responsibilities, all the time failing to recognise the cumulative impact of certain obligations and activities on her mental health and wellbeing.

Osaka's experience played out, in real-time, an extremely public microcosm of social anxiety highlighting not only the interactions and situations that cause distress but also the social conditions and structures that exacerbate and sustain social fears and lead to further isolation, marginalisation and exclusion from key areas of social life. Osaka demonstrated a profound exercise of self-care by pre-empting stressors and taking steps to mitigate and alleviate her anxiety; steps that would have enabled her to undertake other key aspects of her job, most notably competing in the tournament. However, her much-maligned decision drew not only scrutiny and criticism but public comparisons with her peers, responses likely to fuel already persistent negative self-evaluations. To add insult to injury, the official French Open Twitter account appeared to mock Osaka. Tweeting alongside photos of other athletes engaged in media appearances, the caption: "They understood the assignment".[1] This too chimed with opinions from other athletes who, disagreeing with Osaka's media "boycott", stated that media obligations are simply "part of the job" and that "we know what we sign up for as professional tennis players" (Oxley, 2021). The FTF also chastised her decision as "detrimental or injurious to the grand slam tournaments" while journalists argued that the "self-imposed barrier" placed between Osaka and the media set "a very dangerous precedent" one that would "be a hugely destructive and massive commercial blow to everyone in the sport" (Castle, 2021). The negative response fuelled stigma about and misrepresentations of Osaka's competence and her commitment to the sport with her overall actions cast as a sign of personal weakness or laziness (Kumble, Diddi and Bien-Aimé, 2022). Right-wing journalists labelled her a "spoiled brat" and "narcissistic", accusing her of "cynical exploitation of mental health to silence the media" (Morgan, 2021). It should be noted that this was the first press conference Osaka missed in seven years and, as she stated herself, it would be hard to "imagine another profession where a consistent attendance record [...] would be so harshly scrutinised" (Osaka, 2021).

As these events unfolded, they demonstrated that there remains a critical lack of understanding about social anxiety, whether that be in sport, in the media or by the general public. It served as an unfortunate yet timely reminder of the numerous personal and (small "p") political reasons underlying why I have continued to research and write about social anxiety for the last decade, exploring people's lived experiences through a human-geographical lens to understand better the everyday interactions, sites and settings that exacerbate and sustain social fears and social anxieties. Most people's experiences are, of course, rarely as public as Osaka's, with their ongoing attempts to manage and navigate daily life largely going unseen and unnoticed. To this end, this book is an attempt to examine social anxiety through the words of those for whom significant aspects of daily life are impacted by it, to create a more sympathetic and authentic rendering of the socially anxious life, and indeed – sympathetically, not in an "exposing" manner – make it "a little more" visible to others.

Note

1 A phrase popular on social media to acknowledge someone has done an exceptional job or exceeded expectations.

References

Castle, A. (2021) 'Naomi Osaka's French Open decision sets a dangerous precedent', *Metro*, 28 May. https://metro.co.uk/2021/05/28/naomi-osakas-silence-at-french-open-sets-a-dangerous-precedent-14664225/ (Accessed: 21 June 2023).

Daugherty, P. (2021) 'Paul Daugherty: Naomi Osaka is honest, thoughtful and could help many other athletes', *The Enquirer*, 17 August. https://www.cincinnati.com/story/sports/2021/08/17/naomi-osaka-cincinnati-tennis-star-could-help-other-athletes-column/8156280002/ (Accessed: 23 June 2023).

Kumble, S., Diddi, P., and Bien-Aimé, S. (2022) '"Your Strength Is Inspirational": How Naomi Osaka's Twitter Announcement Destigmatizes Mental Health Disclosures', *Communication & Sport*. https://doi.org/10.1177/21674795221124584

Morgan, P. (2021) 'Narcissistic Naomi's exploitation of mental health', *Mail Online*, 31 May.https://www.dailymail.co.uk/news/article-9636993/PIERS-MORGAN-Narcissistic-Naomis-cynical-exploitation-mental-health-silence-media.html (Accessed: 7 August 2023).

NaomiOsaka大坂なおみ [@naomiosaka] (2021) 'https://t.co/LN2ANnoAYD', *Twitter*. https://twitter.com/naomiosaka/status/1399422304854188037 (Accessed: 21 June 2023).

Osaka, N. (2021) Naomi Osaka: 'It's O.K. Not to Be O.K.', *Time*. https://time.com/6077128/naomi-osaka-essay-tokyo-olympics/ (Accessed: 21 June 2023).

Oxley, S. (2021) 'What might Osaka's media boycott achieve?', *BBC Sport*. https://www.bbc.com/sport/tennis/57270276 (Accessed: 25 June 2023).

Roland-Garros (2021) *Statement from Grand Slam tournaments regarding Naomi Osaka - Roland-Garros - The 2021 Roland-Garros Tournament official site.* https://www.rolandgarros.com/en-us/article/statement-from-grand-slam-tournaments-regarding-naomi-osaka (Accessed: 30 September 2021).

Tuakli-Wosornu, Y.A. and Darling-Hammond, K. (2022) 'Unapologetic refusals: Black women in sport model a modern mental health promotion strategy', *Lancet Regional Health - Americas*, 15, p. 100342. https://doi.org/10.1016/j.lana.2022.100342

Acknowledgements

This book would not have come to fruition without the vast circle of people who, whether they realise it or not, have supported me and spurred me on over the years. I wish to express my gratitude towards a number of people.

First and foremost, this book would not have been possible without the people who participated in this research. I am grateful beyond measure for your candour, generosity and willingness to discuss your experiences with me. I am continually in awe of your ability to put the often-indescribable motions of social anxiety into words. Your stories have helped shape the direction of this research and my own understanding of social anxiety. I hope to have done your words justice.

I also gratefully acknowledge the School of Geographical and Earth Sciences at the University of Glasgow, which has been my academic home in numerous capacities over the last 15 years. This research, and all of the opportunities afforded to me, would not have been possible without the financial support of the Economic and Social Research Council for funding the PhD Scholarship (+3) (Award Number: ES/J500136/1); the Scottish Graduate School of Social Sciences for funding an Overseas Institutional Visit (OIV) to Simon Fraser University (SFU), Burnaby; and the Economic and Social Research Council Post-Doctoral Fellowship (Award Number: ES/V0118391).

I have worked on most of this book "outside" of academia and so, I am extremely grateful to the Society of Authors, who funded a generous Authors' Foundation grant that enabled me to prioritise this writing project, lifting the financial burden of precarious and unemployment and inspiring some much-needed confidence to see it through to the end.

This book unfolded during and after my time at the University of Glasgow, and I have been continuously supported and gently encouraged by wonderful colleagues and mentors. I do not have the words to convey the immense gratitude I have for the intellectual curiosity and generosity of Chris Philo, you saw something valuable in this research over a decade ago and have steadfastly championed it, and me, ever since. To Cheryl McGeachan, thank you for being a constant source of encouragement, support, reassurance and giggles over the years. I am so grateful for your ever-kind and thoughtful encouragement of my work. I am also extremely grateful to Hester Parr for your wonderful mentorship during a difficult pandemic-impacted fellowship, for your ongoing kindness and support and for helping me get this whole endeavour off the ground. I must also thank Sara MacKian for planting the seed that the thesis should be developed into a monograph and for helpful feedback on proposals and chapters alike; and Gavin Andrews for casting a helpful eye over some of this material. To Paul Kingsbury, for hosting my OIV to SFU and your guidance in all things psycho-analysis. Finally, to Natalie Prevost, for being an academic eye outside of geography, I am so grateful for your commitment to reading through the majority of this book and, most of all, your friendship.

I have lived in many places while writing both the original thesis and this book and I am grateful to a beautiful network of friends who have supported me over the years with glasses of wine, spaces to write, hikes and adventures. In Vancouver: Rachel, Kensie, Hossein, Tom and all those who were a part of the daily machinations of "The Store" and beyond. I'm beyond grateful for your friendship. In Bangkok: Kat, David, Thanan, Elizabeth, Joe, Chrissy, Mike, Jan, Katherine and "adventuring crews" new and old, thank you for the coffee breaks, pastries, soup curry and adventures that have kept me going throughout. At home, in Scotland: Kerrie, Vikki, Sadie, Sarah and Laurie, I miss you all. To the lockdown lunch crew: Fran, Eleanor, Tom and Phil, thank you for being there every day during the pandemic. You guys really kept me going! A special mention to Nicola and Maricela, for your friendship and supportive podcasts over the years; and to Kenny, for the lengthy chats and rants at all hours about life with social anxiety – I'm very grateful for you, pal!

To my family for supporting all of my whims and endeavours in life. My wee maw, you deserve so much more than a few lines of thanks here but thank you for everything you have done and continue to do, for all of us. Dad, for your unwavering belief in me and always being proud of my achievements. My big brothers, Stephen and Alan, and to Naoko, a special thank you for your keen interest in my work.

Last, but by no means least, I owe endless amounts of thanks to Mitchell, I am not sure words are enough for the love and patience you have shown me throughout this endeavour. Thank you for being a sounding board, a proof-reader, for building me up, talking me down and continually reminding me, "You've got this!" Thank you does not seem enough, but I am beyond grateful for you.

1 Introduction

Introduction

Life with social anxiety is kind of empty and hopeless at times. My anxiety tells me that I'm not good enough, that I will fail, embarrass myself, be laughed at, be humiliated or ignored, and then be rejected by others. How do you live in a world when you are scared of other people? When you're scared to interact or connect with others for fear of what they will think of you? It always looks so easy from the outside looking in but it often feels like there's an invisible wall between me and everyone else. It's as if there's a barrier between me and the life I should be living.

Throughout my life, I've been thought of as shy or introverted. People have said I come across as aloof, even rude and arrogant because I keep myself to myself and don't really engage in conversation, but I'm not. I am painfully anxious when I am around other people and painfully aware of myself. I'm anxious about the minute details of every interaction. I pick apart facial expressions, tones of voice, body movements, what I said, how I said it, and the level of eye contact I made, and convince myself that somehow I made that person feel uncomfortable, or they will think I'm stupid or weird or awkward. My anxiety goes through the roof sometimes and I have to spend hours, sometimes days, calming myself down again. I replay moments in my head over and over and over and deal with intrusive thoughts about things that happened years ago.

And it really takes its toll, you know? Not being able to do the 'simple' things that most people don't even think about like, answer the door or make a phone call, take the bus, cross the street, order a coffee, eat in public, all because of a crippling fear that people will notice me and judge me. I just don't want to be seen or have any attention drawn to me. I prepare excessively for every situation in advance. I plan what I'll say and try to account for every eventuality. It is exhausting. Failing that, I avoid situations entirely.

My social anxiety has gotten worse over the years, and I have slowly withdrawn from social life. Most of my days are spent at home. I am

DOI: 10.4324/9781003206880-1

really a shell of a person. I've missed out on a lot of life experiences. I dropped out of university, I don't have a job, never dated anyone, don't have a close circle of friends, or hobbies. I've missed weddings, birthdays, funerals and memorable events. Every day feels the same. I feel like I exist but I'm not actually living. Seeing everyone and everything around me grow and change while I remain stagnant really puts a strain on my self-esteem and any ambition I might have once had. It's hard to build any kind of momentum for life. I feel pretty worthless about that.

If anything, I hope people are able to understand what it's like to live with social anxiety, just a little bit – GOD I would NOT want anyone to have to live like this, scared of the world, scared of other people, feeling like you don't belong anywhere, feeling uncomfortable in your own skin! … but I'd hope they could connect with some part of it and realise how much it consumes our lives.[1]

This book is about the lived experiences of social anxiety. Therefore, it feels appropriate to begin with the words of those who contributed their personal stories and experiences to this research. Their words have not only nurtured my own distinctive socio-spatial understanding of social anxiety and shaped the direction of this research immeasurably, they have also, more importantly, elucidated in stark detail the complexity of their anxious worlds. Throughout, I have given priority to their words, centring the particular and the subjective content of how social anxiety is lived with and through in order to emphasise that anxious distress carries diverse meanings for different individuals in the context of their daily lives.

Motivation and aims

The motivation for writing this book is both personal and academic. Throughout my life, and with varying levels of disruption and intensity, I have lived with social anxiety. At its most disruptive, I felt overwhelming fear and anxiety about being in public, I found myself avoiding situations that made me anxious, I had to take time out of my final year of my undergraduate degree at university and I felt isolated and alienated from others. I spent months searching online trying to find an explanation, simply trying to make sense of what I was experiencing. Inevitably, social anxiety appeared in the search results, but the information available at the time did not resonate with me. The explanations I found online for the anxieties I was experiencing were removed from the social contexts and environments that I was experiencing them in. Perhaps owing to a love of human geography and being engaged in "geographical thought" at university at this time, I could not shake the idea that there was something *inherently spatial* about what I was experiencing particularly as my perceptions of and interactions with my surroundings changed; I felt isolated and disconnected from others; I was safe *here* but not *there*; *my world* had gotten smaller. My anxiety was mapped onto, threaded through and starting to affect the social fabric and relations that "made up" my everyday life, but those aspects, ones so central to my experience, were entirely missing from the information available online, in mental health literature and in conversations with doctors and therapists. Nothing seemed to capture, and no one seemed to be addressing, what I did not have terminology for then but what I now understand to be, its geography.

This crucial absence led me to the academic motivation: to understand the social and spatial underpinnings of social anxiety. I began to map out the early coordinates of this research, assuming there would be a strong foundation of experiential literature for me to draw upon, however, I found the reality to be quite the opposite. Research that engaged with – substantively, properly listening to – lived experiences of social anxiety was, and remains, scarce. On the most fundamental level, I wanted to know if other people experienced and managed their social anxiety *socially* or, indeed, *spatially*; and whether reframing their experiences in such a way could just possibly provide some therapeutic benefits. As a result, this book is based on an ESRC[2]-funded PhD research project (Boyle, 2019),[3] a project book-ended by a Masters by Research dissertation (Boyle, 2011) and an ESRC-funded Post-Doctoral Fellowship.[4] The various iterations of this research have sought to explore the lived experiences and social geographies of people living with social anxiety, unearthing and critically inspecting the social and spatial contingencies that shape the experience and expression of anxious distress. It set out to examine the influence that social anxiety has on daily life and how it is implicated in a variety of social interactions, sites and settings. With that, this work has been concerned with people's diverse and adverse social experiences, the bodily responses and emotional intensities they provoke, how they ameliorate and navigate them and how they understand and make sense of their experiences in the course of their daily lives. In considering the geographical potentials of social anxiety and the personal geographies that underpin its experience, this book makes three related but specific contributions.

First, it provides detailed accounts of the everyday lives of people living with social anxiety. The primary aim here is to understand *precisely* what it is like to live with social anxiety, retrieving the experiences that profoundly disrupt a person's sense of being in the world and shaping their interactions with and within it. Research on lived experiences of social anxiety is extremely limited. We know very little about the personal, relational and social dimensions of this innately *social* condition and what it *feels* like to experience profound anxiety about a world shared with others. While these stories are contextualised into broader academic discussions in the geographies of health and wellbeing and beyond, they stand in their own right as experiential knowledges, offering contextual and nuanced understandings of the "everydayness" of anxious distress.

Second, it challenges and nuances overly reductive accounts of social anxiety. Current perspectives are fairly one-dimensional, focusing predominantly on the cognitive and physiological symptoms of disorder with ongoing attempts to attribute these symptoms to underlying pathological mechanisms or biological markers of disease (Caldiroli *et al.*, 2023). Such approaches reduce experience to quantifiable events ignoring the everyday contexts of a person's subjective life world. Isolating symptoms from their social and emotional contexts strips the individual of the personal, social, spatial and cultural significance – the *meaning* – of their anxious distress and failing to recognise this reductive move effaces the embodied and socially situated nature of distress as well as the contexts in which it is shaped, exacerbated and also alleviated. My approach, in contrast, aims to cut across the boundaries of what is considered "normal" versus "pathological", challenging the continued medicalisation of anxious distress. It does so not to negate the disruptive and unsettling capacities of anxiety or negate the debilitating impacts it has on a person's life, nor to minimise a person's experience by rendering it as something more akin to embarrassment or shyness, albeit these aspects do indeed feature in the experience of social anxiety - they cannot capture it in its totality. Instead, it serves to locate a middle ground, recognising that, rather than biological fact, anxious distress is instead *mediated* by biological factors – expressed physiologically or behaviourally – and embodied by people situated in their relational and material worlds.

Third, building from the first two aims, this work advances a novel conceptualisation of social anxiety as a social and spatial phenomenon, one that can be better understood by paying attention to the everyday spaces, material conditions and bodily intensities at play in the daily lives of those experiencing it. Anxious experiences are embroiled in a complex set of social and contextual relationships profoundly shaped by our social and spatial surroundings. And there is a double relationship at work here: one where, on one axis, anxieties shape the perception or experience a person has of/in a particular place or space, but where, on a second axis, interactions, sites or settings, integral to social life, shape the intensities and contours of anxious experience.

Overall, this book explores how we can better understand social anxiety and support those living with it. It also aims to generate new knowledges about people's anxious experiences and the broader implications for their health and wellbeing, and perhaps more importantly, their very sense of being. I hope that this book can go some way to remedy the present absences in extent research and thinking around social anxiety, and thereby foster a newer emerging field of research that can indeed take seriously and prioritise lived experiences of social anxiety.

A note on terminology

Throughout this text, a number of terms are used to refer to the concept and experience of social anxiety. I will predominantly use the term "social anxiety" when addressing the personal geographies of people's experiences, but I should outline some of the conditions and contexts in which other terms are employed to designate aspects of the anxious experience.

First, social anxiety disorder or SAD[5] is used to designate the clinical category of disorder as outlined by the American Psychiatric Association's

Diagnostic and Statistical Manual of Mental Disorders (DSM) (Chapter 2) or when participants who find utility in the term explicitly refer to their experiences as such. Second, social anxiety disorder was previously known as "social phobia", a term more commonly used in scholarly and clinical literature pre-2014 (Lloyd, 2006) and still utilised by proponents of particular interpersonal models (Stravynski, 2007, 2014). In many ways, social phobia is a more encompassing term that extends beyond the narrow focus on the symptom of anxiety, but in what follows social phobia will only be used to refer to early clinical definitions of the disorder (Chapter 2) and where other research and participants explicitly employ the term. I have therefore settled on the term "social anxiety", acknowledging as well that not everyone (including many of the participants in this research) has sought or received a formal diagnosis of social anxiety *disorder* from a medical professional (Chapter 5). Participants – whether or not they have received a diagnosis – tend to drop the "disorder" when considering or relating to their own lived experience, whether out of ease or maybe even resistance to being described as "disordered". It is the terminology used most often by participants in this study; it is the term or concept that they research online and elsewhere, about which they communicate with others and through which they understand their fears and anxieties about social situations. Finally, with regard to advancing a social and spatial understanding of social anxiety – one that views social anxiety as more than an innate problem within the individual and seeks to account for the wider personal and social geographies that enable social anxiety to thrive – and also to disentangle social anxiety from rigid medicalised frameworks, other terms are occasionally deployed, such as anxious distress, social fears and emotional distress to refer to various aspects of the anxious experience or social anxiety in its entirety.

Researching social anxiety

Despite the personal motivation for this research, this project is not autoethnographic in nature and I have refrained from situating my personal experiences alongside those of research participants throughout, but unavoidably, my experiences have influenced the research design, methodological approach and then, analysis and interpretation of the data. Solely first-person perspectives in academic work have flourished in recent years, particularly around mental health (Costa *et al.*, 2012; Callard, 2014; Bertilsdotter Rosqvist *et al.*, 2023) offering nuanced accounts that centre ambivalence about and resistance to mental health systems and research agendas as well as enabling people to take (back) control of their own narratives. I disclosed my experiences of social anxiety to research participants from the outset to position myself as "someone familiar", which helped to establish some commonalities and build rapport, trust and mutual understanding with research participants (Gair, 2012). However, I did not want to complicate, or even "muddy", participants experiences with my own. I have discussed how personal and professional worlds intertwine in simultaneously beneficial and uncomfortable ways, as well as the challenges and advantages of this insider-outsider position, elsewhere (Philo, Boyle and Lucherini, 2021).

My experiences did, however, equip me with some insights into the anxious experience, which helped me anticipate and navigate some of the challenges people may face when it comes to the research encounter, which is, in and of itself, a social interaction. People with social anxiety often face immense difficulties and distress during social interactions and so the traditional social-scientific research encounter, which prioritises direct fieldwork and in-person data collection, is likely to present considerable challenges for exploring the geographies of the anxious experience. My research was sensitive to the likelihood that individuals may experience distress during, or might actively avoid participating in, research involving face-to-face or verbal methods of communication. This is not to say that people with social anxiety are incapable of participating in in-person research methods, as other research has demonstrated (Scott, 2004; McCarthy, 2014), but it gives due consideration to the fact that many do struggle with social interactions and that anxieties may be further aggravated by a number of factors, including the nature of the research encounter, the position of the researcher, power relations between researcher and researched, and aspects of non-verbal communication such as social cues, eye contact and body language. Therefore, an essential component of the research was to ensure participants did not experience any unnecessary distress as a result of their participation. Consequently, the research was conducted primarily online using a multi-method approach, that is, a predominantly qualitative online survey and online semi-structured interviews on a text-based messaging platform. A small number of participants opted to participate via telephone interviews due to preference or lack of technology.

At the time this research was conducted, there were a number of misplaced assumptions about online research, in particular regarding the perceived difficulty in securing detailed representations of experience, the kind central to this research, and more broadly, its capacity to gather in-depth information about the complexity of people's social and spatial worlds. The extent to which these remain, or have indeed been challenged, as a result of the COVID-19 pandemic, which necessitated an immediate shift to online or remote methodologies for the vast majority of researchers globally, remains to be seen, but I offer some reflections on how a carefully considered online approach can be implemented to enrich geographical inquiry and to elaborate on what this approach provides for the inclusion of people living with social anxiety.

Research participants were invited to answer an online questionnaire via two UK-based online support forums for people with social anxiety – one of which has since stopped operating[6] – and a UK-based charity supporting people with anxiety more generally. Recruitment, via these channels, provides an avenue to reach socially "remote" populations who would otherwise have been difficult to access and who may have lacked the offline services and communities required for support. In addition, I was conscious that delving into and sharing acutely personal experiences of social anxiety may be upsetting or cause distress that I would not be able to see or respond to (Bowker and Tuffin, 2004), and so recruitment through such channels was important as it meant that participants were at least be aware of, and hence have potential access to, peer support and other informational and therapeutic resources, even if they were not actively engaged in these communities.[7]

The first stage of the research process involved designing and implementing a predominantly qualitative online survey to gather experiential accounts about people's lives with social anxiety. It also gathered some basic biographical information and descriptive statistics. Surveys are often considered essential to the geographer's toolkit for gathering information about the characteristics, perceptions and attitudes of a given population (Cloke *et al.*, 2004; McLafferty, 2010; McGuirk and O'Neill, 2016). In the geographies of health and wellbeing, more qualitative-leaning surveys have been used as part of multi-method studies to gather data on the health experiences, behaviours and practices on potentially sensitive topics and with vulnerable and/or hard-to-reach groups, including diabetes (Lucherini, 2020), epilepsy (Smith, 2012) and neurodiversity and autism (Henderson *et al.*, 2014; Kenna, 2023).

With online research, there are preconceptions about qualitative surveys and the depth and richness of qualitative data that can be produced compared to other qualitative methods (Braun *et al.*, 2021). For example, de Vaus (2013) argues that surveys do not allow for the complexities and contradictions of experience to be adequately portrayed. However, the survey approach was an inherently positive aspect of the research design, strengthening rather than hindering the quality and quantity of the resulting data. The online and anonymous mode helped to facilitate participation while the asynchronous nature provided an environment where participants had the time, space and privacy to consider their responses. Given that many individuals with social anxiety find the proximity and immediacy of in-person communications distressing, the survey enabled the subtleties and nuances of their experience to be expressed in written form, a more comfortable medium of communication for those who are often regularly engaged in writing about and discussing their experiences in online forums.

At the end of the survey, participants were invited to participate in a follow-up interview. Semi-structured interviews were conducted with self-selecting survey respondents. Three opted to participate via telephone interviews. The online interviews were conducted in real-time through a (now defunct) online messaging platform, ChatStep. This platform was chosen as it did not require participants to sign up or download any programs or software to their devices. I was able to create password-protected rooms and invite participants via a link, and data was not retained by the website's servers. At the end of the interviews, a transcript of the conversation was immediately available to download, and participants could retain a copy for their own records. The "placing" of interviews was of particular concern given that face-to-face interviews would have been difficult, if not distressing, for many participants. I aimed to make the research design as flexible, inclusive and accessible as possible, offering online text-based interviews in the first instance and discussing other options

on an individual basis. This approach proved to be beneficial as many participants demonstrated concerns about face-to-face or telephone interactions in
their remarks at the end of the initial survey. Several participants stated explicitly that they would only participate further via online methods:

> I'd much prefer online, as I struggle to answer phone calls, but I would be
> happy to take part in a follow up interview online.
>
> (Olivia, QR)

> I'm willing to do it online, not in person or via Skype.
>
> (Molly, QR)

For one participant, despite the anonymity offered by the online environment,
the immediacy of a synchronous exchange was as distressing as face-to-face
interactions:

> Even the thought of an interview online terrifies me. I may not be of any
> further use to you but I will give you my email address. I can always
> decline can't I?
>
> (Tina, QR)

I contacted Tina shortly afterwards acknowledging her concerns and providing
more information about the interview process. Unfortunately, I did not receive
a response but the detail with which she initially recorded her experiences in the
survey response has been extremely valuable to the research findings. Three
participants favoured telephone interviews over online. Two (Moira and Nina)
had no anxieties about communicating over the phone and one (Karen) had no
home internet connection or access to a laptop but found the project while
browsing the research listing on the charity's website on her mobile phone.
Both Karen and Nina did not complete the online survey but wanted to share
their experiences via an interview, further cementing the value of maintaining
an open and flexible approach that responded to the needs of participants.

Finally, throughout this book, all participants have been assigned pseud-
onyms and I have indicated whether the source of their data is from questionnaire responses (QR) or interview responses (IR). Participants' words are
presented verbatim, including swearing (as it often captures the frustrations
and exasperations inherent in people's experiences), the use of slang and local
idiosyncrasies in language (particularly between myself and other Scottish participants) and the use of acronyms and emojis commonplace in electronic
forms of communication (as forms of body language and gestures missing
from the text-based nature of our communications). I have also presented text
in the format it was given, for example, bullet points used in the online questionnaire and line breaks in the online interview material capture the individual and sequential nature of messages. Questionnaire and interview material
has occasionally been edited for length and clarity. Where information has

been added for clarity is indicated by "[ ]" brackets around the text; omitted information is indicated by "[...]" throughout.

Structure of this book

This book is structured into seven main chapters, two conceptual and five empirical, and a final conclusion, which will provide a summary and point to some recommendations for future research and practice. Each of the analysis chapters focuses on a different spatial experience and can be read independently of the others. That said, each of these chapters does build on the preceding one and, when put altogether, they provide an in-depth understanding of how people with social anxiety experience and navigate their social and spatial worlds.

Chapter 2 offers a concise historical exploration of social anxiety's evolution from its initial recognition to its inclusion as a "disorder" in the American Psychiatric Association's Diagnostic and Statistical Manual of Mental Disorders. It highlights the subtle yet influential shifts in its classification that defined it as a psychological disorder. The chapter also acknowledges the limited existing sociological research on social anxiety, shyness and related social fears, providing essential context for the subsequent in-depth examination of the geographical dimensions of social anxiety that form the substance of this book. This historical and sociological overview serves as a valuable foundation for understanding the complex background of social anxiety's conceptualisation and its societal implications. Chapter 3 attends to the conceptual underpinnings of the research, providing an overview of the relevant literatures in the geographies of health and wellbeing and related fields. Drawing on humanistic and post-humanist insights that enrich geographical approaches to health, illness and wellbeing, it introduces the core concepts that underpin this work: spatial dimensions, temporal aspects and embodied experiences. Chapter 4 explores the emotional and affective "intensities" of social anxiety in order to examine the various ways in which social anxiety is embodied and enacted as people orientate their social and spatial worlds. Through the intensities of participants' experiences, this chapter considers the force and form of social anxiety and how, materially and discursively, these manifestations texture participants' everyday lives. Chapter 5 examines the diagnostic journeys of social anxiety. First, addressing online spaces as the first point of contact for people seeking information about their mental health. Then, attending to the various critical junctures at which people seek a diagnosis (or not), it examines the role played by various medical and therapeutic spaces. This chapter explores how individuals obtain and make use of a diagnosis within, alongside or outwith[8] medical treatment pathways. It pays attention to how medical practice and spaces not only shape the experience of diagnosis, but also lay the groundwork for the course of treatment, care and "recovery". Chapters 6 explores the spatial contingencies of living with social anxiety in order to map the disrupted and the disruptive geographies of anxious experience. It pays attention to the formative spaces of home and work, taking into consideration the complexity of physical, material and socio-spatial factors that comprise these everyday spaces and the practices that emerge through them. This inquiry reveals some of the continuous or repeated negative experiences embedded in people's everyday lives, relationships and spaces – particularly those potentially damaging to their overall wellbeing. Chapter 7 deepens the accounts from Chapter 6, acknowledging that the "progression" of social anxiety is associated with increased socio-spatial isolation as patterns of social interaction change and public space is encountered with greater difficulty or avoided completely. Social and interpersonal relationships are intimately tied with the "self", thus the physical and emotional need to distance oneself from these anxiety-inducing objects is complex, often distressing and increasingly isolating. This chapter explores how uncertain interpersonal worlds are compounded by an overwhelming fear of humiliation, embarrassment and rejection that has the potential to lead to avoidance, loneliness, isolation and a broader withdrawal from social and public spaces. This deeper examination of people's worlds uncovers the complexity in, and limitations placed on, everyday social life. Chapter 8 discusses everyday coping strategies with reference to geographical debates on habit. It considers how habit simultaneously captures (un)reflective modes of being-in-the-world and the foreboding, repetitive and disruptive capacity of anxious distress experienced by people as they attempt to adapt to, negotiate and manage everyday life with social anxiety.

Notes

1 This introductory section is a creative rendition of the responses of five participants, each highlighting a significant way in which social anxiety has impacted their life.
2 Economic and Social Research Council offers funding for postgraduate and post-doctoral research in the UK.
3 Award number: ES/J500136/1
4 Award number: ES/V0118391
5 Not to be confused with Seasonal Affective Disorder.
6 This highlights some of the issues surrounding the lack of formal and accessible support for people experiencing social anxiety and the burden this places on user-led online communities especially those funded, managed and maintained by a sole or small groups of individual(s).
7 Participants were also provided with region-specific information on mental health support services at the beginning and end of the survey and on the research information sheets provided for the follow-up interviews.
8 Scottish. Meaning "outside of".

References

Bertilsdotter Rosqvist, H. et al. (2023) 'Naming ourselves, becoming neurodivergent scholars', *Disability & Society*, pp. 1–20. Available at: https://doi.org/10.1080/0968759 9.2023.2271155

Bowker, N. and Tuffin, K. (2004) 'Using the Online Medium for Discursive Research About People With Disabilities', *Social Science Computer Review*, 22(2), pp. 228–241. Available at: https://doi.org/10.1177/0894439303262561

Boyle, L. (2011) *Lived experiences of social anxiety disorder*. Unpublished Masters by Research Dissertation. University of Glasgow.

Boyle, L. (2019) *The social and anticipatory geographies of social anxiety*. Unpublished PhD Thesis. University of Glasgow. Available at: http://theses.gla.ac.uk/74345/ (Accessed: 4 August 2021).

Braun, V. et al. (2021) 'The online survey as a qualitative research tool', *International Journal of Social Research Methodology*, 24(6), pp. 641–654. Available at: https://doi.org/10.1080/13645579.2020.1805550

Caldiroli, A. et al. (2023) 'Candidate Biological Markers for Social Anxiety Disorder: A Systematic Review', *International Journal of Molecular Sciences*, 24(1), p. 835. Available at: https://doi.org/10.3390/ijms24010835

Callard, F. (2014) 'Psychiatric diagnosis: the indispensability of ambivalence', *Journal of Medical Ethics*, 40(8), pp. 526–530. Available at: https://doi.org/10.1136/medethics-2013-101763

Cloke, P. et al. (2004) *Practising Human Geography*. London. Available at: https://doi.org/10.4135/9781446221235

Costa, L. et al. (2012) '"Recovering our Stories": A Small Act of Resistance', *Studies in Social Justice*, 6(1), pp. 85–101. Available at: https://doi.org/10.26522/ssj.v6i1.1070

de Vaus, D. (2013) *Surveys In Social Research*. 6th edn. London: Routledge. Available at: https://doi.org/10.4324/9780203519196

Gair, S. (2012) 'Feeling Their Stories: Contemplating Empathy, Insider/Outsider Positionings, and Enriching Qualitative Research', *Qualitative Health Research*, 22(1), pp. 134–143. Available at: https://doi.org/10.1177/1049732311420580

Henderson, V. et al. (2014) 'Hacking the master code: cyborg stories and the boundaries of autism', *Social & Cultural Geography*, 15(5), pp. 504–524. Available at: https://doi.org/10.1080/14649365.2014.898781

Kenna, T. (2023) 'Neurodiversity in the city: Exploring the complex geographies of belonging and exclusion in urban space', *The Geographical Journal*, 189(2), pp. 370–382. Available at: https://doi.org/10.1111/geoj.12512

Lloyd, S. (2006) 'The Clinical Clash over Social Phobia: The Americanization of French Experiences?', *BioSocieties*, 1(2), pp. 229–249. Available at: https://doi.org/10.1017/S1745855206060042

Lucherini, M. (2020) 'Spontaneity and serendipity: Space and time in the lives of people with diabetes', *Social Science & Medicine*, 245, p. 112723. Available at: https://doi.org/10.1016/j.socscimed.2019.112723

McCarthy, C. (2014) *Social Anxiety: Personal Narratives on Journeys to Recovery*. London, UK: University of East London.

McGuirk, P.M. and O'Neill, P. (2016) 'Using questionnaires in qualitative human geography', in I. Hay (ed.) *Qualitative Research Methods in Human Geography*. London: Oxford University Press, pp. 246–273.

McLafferty, S. (2010) 'Conducting Questionnaire Surveys', in N. Clifford, S. French, and G. Valentine (eds) *Key Methods in Human Geography*. London: SAGE Publications, pp. 77–88.

Philo, C., Boyle, L. and Lucherini, M. (2021) 'Creative Methods for Human Geographers', in N.V. Benzon et al. (eds) *Creative Methods for Human Geographers*. SAGE Publications, pp. 35–48.

Scott, S. (2004) 'Researching shyness: a contradiction in terms?', *Qualitative Research*, 4(1), pp. 91–105. Available at: https://doi.org/10.1177/1468794104041109

Smith, N. (2012) 'Embodying brainstorms: the experiential geographies of living with epilepsy', *Social & Cultural Geography*, 13(4), pp. 339–359. Available at: https://doi.org/10.1080/14649365.2012.683806

Stravynski, A. (2007) *Fearing Others: The Nature and Treatment of Social Phobia.* Cambridge University Press.

Stravynski, A. (2014) *Social Phobia: An Interpersonal Approach.* Cambridge University Press.

2 The medicalisation of anxious distress

Introduction

Before turning to the geographical substance of this book, it is useful to provide a brief ethnography of social anxiety and its emergence as a "disorder".[1] Despite its early status as a "neglected disorder" (Liebowitz *et al.*, 1985), the history of social anxiety disorder, and its precursor social phobia, is contentious and complex. Tracing its history from the earliest identifications to its induction into the American Psychiatric Association's (APA) Diagnostic and Statistical Manual of Mental Disorders[2] Third Edition (DSM-III), and into subsequent iterations, illuminates several small but significant changes to its classification that shaped its status as a "disorder". The wider implications of these changes are considered. Then, this chapter briefly outlines the small body of existing research on social anxiety, and related concepts of shyness and social fears, within more sociological-leaning fields.

A "neglected disorder"

The phenomena that manifest in the lived experience of social anxiety are not new, but what has changed significantly is the focus and "emphasis" on particular signs, symptoms, behaviours and contexts of anxiety, the various "permutations and combinations" with which a person may present in order to obtain a specific diagnosis, the thresholds, and most significantly, "their social meanings" (Berrios, 1999 p. 83). The modern concept of social anxiety disorder as a diagnosable clinical entity has developed slowly and episodically over the course of the 20th century,[3] attracting relatively short periods of intense attention (and controversy) with longer, sustained periods of apparent neglect. One of the earliest formal classifications pertaining to phobias of social situations can be found in the work[4] of French psychiatrist Pierre Janet, who coined the term social phobia in 1903 to designate a class of situational phobias. The defining features of which were a fear of others, being in the company of others, being visible to others, being in public and of having to act in public. Janet outlines four categories of phobias (*'les phobies'*): of the body, of objects, of ideas and of situations. The scope of the latter is extremely broad and further

DOI: 10.4324/9781003206880-2

broken down into phobias of physical situations, for example, claustrophobia or agoraphobia; and social situations, for example, erythrophobia (fear of blushing) and dysmorphophobia (fixation on, and anxiety about, personal features, figure and movements), as well as fear and avoidance of social contracts including marriage and employment. While Janet considered the root cause of social phobias – "psychasthenia" – to be a distinct and serious disease, Valsiner and van der Veer (2000, p. 119) argue that he also "resisted any attempt at explaining personality by exclusive reference to biological, or associational, findings" and instead sought to understand "the individual acting within a complex social environment" (p. 124).

Thus, Janet details cases of people who do not want to see anyone or enter public life; who are fearful of how their physical appearance, personality or behaviours will be perceived and judged by others; of a young women named Claire who, as a result of perceived personal "defects", says that it *"mieux vaudrait mourir*[5] [would be better to die]" (Janet, 1903, p. 48) than to go outside, dine in a restaurant or get married; of a teacher, forced to give up his job because he could not attend classes or meetings for fear of wetting himself in public; a telegraph operator who can no longer work due to a fear of the post office; of a man in his thirties, living alone in such abject fear of being heard by his neighbours and of his mother visiting unexpectedly that he contemplates suicide; of people who are unable to write, play piano or work in front of others, purchase a train ticket or ask for directions; who are unable to walk into a room where others are present, even at home, and those who are afraid to speak or meet another's gaze for fear of blushing, stuttering or embarrassing themselves. Such cases vividly illustrate how social anxiety can severely hamper not only the interactions, relationships and activities that make up daily life but also individuals' aspirations, vocations and passions. Crucially, Janet's focus centres precisely around the interactions, relations and spaces that comprise daily life. He notes that for *"les phobiques"* [the phobics]:

> *La rue est [...] le symbole de l'isolement et de la lutte, c'est la vie publique oppose à la vie privée [...] c'est dans la rue qu'on les regarde, qu'on les surveille,' qu'on les critique [...] c'est dans la rue qu'on est exposé à toutes sortes d'accidents qui n'arrivent pas chez soi.*
>
> [The road is the symbol of isolation and struggle, it is public life opposed to private life [...] it is in the street that they are looked at, they are watched, they are criticised [...] it is on the road that you are exposed to all kinds of accidents that do not happen at home.]

> (1903, p. 582)

Consequently, Janet notes that "[c]*ette crainte constante à chaque instant réalisée devient [...] un supplice* [the constant fear at every moment becomes a torment]" (1903, p. 214), causing a person to avoid all situations, as well as the social and professional responsibilities that cause emotional pain and distress, and consequently seeking a life of isolation and solitude. Yet, despite the role played by Janet[6] in classifying social phobias in the early 1900s, he is scarcely mentioned in English language histories of the disorder (Lloyd, 2006). Following these early classifications, study of the condition quickly fell out of scholarly fashion and was ultimately neglected for nearly 60 years.

It was not until the late 1950s that the psychiatric classification of social anxieties started to garner attention, particularly amongst British psychiatrists assessing patients diagnosed with various permutations of what was then classified, following the favour of psychoanalysis at this time, as "phobic neurosis". Dixon et al. outlined a number of different anxieties "which occur when the person is concerned with, or anticipates being in, interaction with others" (1957, p. 107) and includes social timidity (e.g. feeling awkward around strangers); fear of loss of control (e.g. fear of fainting or vomiting in public); fear of exhibitionism (e.g. walking past a crowd of people); and fear of revealing inferiority (e.g. being thought of as unintelligent). Later, Marks and Gelder reported a distinction in the age of onset between social anxieties and other phobias, such as agoraphobia, noting that, while the distinction between these two can often seem "rather arbitrary", social anxieties required their own specific designation in the literature (1966, p. 218). Marks (1969) later expanded upon this claim, offering a further distinction between agoraphobia and social phobia by noting that, whereas the former is fear of the masses, the latter is attributed to fear of the individual. He also outlines a cyclical pattern of social phobias: fear of social activities; fear of showing anxiety symptoms that risk exposing oneself to the negative attention of others; leading to a restriction in, or avoidance of, social activities; and impairment in role and social functioning, a cycle which formed the foundation of later cognitive and behavioural models of social anxiety. This early work culminated in the creation of "social phobia" as a clinical entity with its inauguration into the DSM-III in 1980. The intervening years between Marks' work and the DSM witnessed a controversial shift in the theory and practice of mental illness, and a radical transformation in the classification of mental disorders. Despite this, psychiatry was yet to take advantage of social phobia as a "fertile area for psychobiological and clinical investigation" (Liebowitz *et al.*, 1985, p. 729).

The following gives an overview of the changes that have occurred in the diagnostic criteria and terminology of social anxiety over the last five decades. Iterative changes to the diagnostic classification of social anxiety are emblematic of greater shifts in psychiatric theory and practice as well as disputes over the ontological status of mental illness during this period. Prior to publication of the DSM-III, psychiatry was plagued by a "crisis of legitimacy" (Mayes and Horwitz, 2005, pp. 252–253). By discarding the formulations and terminology rooted in the psychoanalytic approaches of the preceding decades, a new psychiatry emerged – one that was empirically based and "atheoretical with regard to aetiology" (APA, 1980, p. 7). These moves were indicative of attempts to obtain objectivity, reliability, validity and accuracy in order to cement psychiatry's position within the scientific community alongside perceived ancillary benefits of stigma reduction and improved access to treatment.[7] However, it has also been argued that they are evidence of the DSM's "plasticity" (Aho, 2010,

p. 5) when it comes to defining the boundaries, thresholds and parameters of diagnostic criteria.

Initially, social phobia was categorised under a subset of "phobic disorders", alongside agoraphobia and simple phobia, with the unifying feature being fear of a specific object, activity or situation that results in avoidance behaviour. In social phobia, this specific concern was:

> A persistent, irrational fear of, and compelling desire to avoid situations in which the individual may be exposed to scrutiny by others. There is also a fear that the individual may behave in a manner that will be humiliating or embarrassing [...] The disturbance is a significant source of distress and is recognized by the individual as excessive or unreasonable.
>
> (American Psychiatric Association, 1980, p. 227)

Generally limited to one phobic situation, the diagnostic criteria centred on performance situations; anxiety-inducing activities including speaking, eating, writing and using public bathrooms. Several years later, DSM-III-Revised expanded the criteria to include "one or more situations" and highlighted the condition's capacity to interfere with social activities, relationships and occupational functioning. Included was a specifier for a generalised sub-type if "the phobic situation includes most social situations" (1987, pp. 241–243). In this case, clinicians were also advised to consider a diagnosis of "avoidant personality disorder" (AvPD), a category intended to account for a broader array of chronic interpersonal anxieties and avoidance. Liebowitz (2010, p. 41) was critical of this distinction, later arguing that "there did not seem to be any empirical basis for" the separation into two distinct disorders. While others justified the separation on account of the "severity of dysfunction and symptomatic distress" (Hummelen *et al.*, 2007, p. 348), Robert Spitzer, Task Force Chair[8] of the DSM-III, notes that "Well, avoidant personality disorder [laughing] is basically identical to social phobia" (Lane, 2022, n.p.). He remarks that AvPD's particular inclusion "was embarrassing [as it] was clear that it was the same as social phobia" yet it was developed by and subsequently included to appease "the personality people" (Lane, 2022). Concern has been expressed about the boundary between the two and whether in fact they can be regarded as two distinct diagnostic categories of disorder, that is, one of "anxiety" and one of "personality" (Widiger, 1992; Huppert *et al.*, 2008), which further feeds into concerns about unreliable and redundant diagnostic categorisations that can result in excessive diagnosis (Tyrer, 2018). DSM-IV (1994) enacted a further change in terminology, inaugurating Social Phobia (Social Anxiety Disorder). In line with wider shifts across psychiatry, the parenthetical addition was thought to more thoroughly represent the clinical situation. This edition also revises the definition to:

> A marked and persistent fear of one or more social or performance situations in which the person is exposed to unfamiliar people or to possible

scrutiny by others. The individual fears that he or she will act in a way (or show anxiety symptoms) that will be humiliating or embarrassing.

(APA 1994, p. 416)

Additionally, individuals no longer needed to "avoid" social situations since even the suffering of having to "endure" any problematic social or performance situation was sufficient for diagnosis. Descriptions also recognised interference with a person's normal routine and ordinary situations. Aho (2010) argues that this slow creep of diagnostic boundaries dramatically widened the parameters for who could be diagnosed with social phobia, evidenced by the number of affected Americans rising from 2.75% to 13% between these DSM publications. Focus was increasingly drawn to both cognitive ideations – for instance, "others will judge them to be anxious, weak, 'crazy', or stupid" – and somatic symptoms, "including palpitations, tremors, sweating, gastrointestinal discomfort, diarrhoea, muscle tension, blushing, confusion" (APA, 1994). That anxiety may manifest in a "situationally-bound or situationally predisposed panic attack" was also highlighted for the first time. Additionally, diagnosis could now be applied to children if the duration of symptoms lasts at least six months. Further qualifiers were added for diagnosing children, including "the anxiety must occur in peer settings and not just during interactions with adults" and "the fear or anxiety may be expressed by crying, tantrums, freezing, clinging, shrinking, or failing to speak in social situations" (1994, p. 417).

DSM-V executed a further change in terminology – switching parenthesis – "Social Anxiety Disorder (Social Phobia)" and expanding the diagnostic criteria to better reflect "a new and broader understanding of the condition in a variety of social situations" (2013b, p. 1). Blushing was noted as a "hallmark physical response" (2013a, p. 204). Fear of being perceived negatively or rejected is expanded to include a fear of offending others. Previously, this "offensive" sub-type was only recognised in "*taijin-kyofu-sho*" (literally, the disorder (*sho*) of fear (*kyofu*) of interpersonal relations (*taijin*)), a Japanese culture-specific syndrome for fear of interpersonal relations, and for which there was previously no direct parallel in Western classification (Tanaka-Matsumi, 1979). More recently, similarities have been drawn between social anxiety disorder, avoidant personality disorder and another Japanese cultural syndrome "*hikikomori*" (literally, to retreat inwards), which is characterised by social withdrawal and prolonged periods of home-bound isolation (Kato, Kanba and Teo, 2018). While this inclusion may suggest attempts to recognise the cultural contexts in which particular social anxieties arise and be indicative of a global approach to mental illness, critics emphasise the "difficulties and potential dangers of applying Western categories, concepts and interventions given the ways that culture shapes illness experience" (Kirmayer and Pedersen, 2014). DSM-V also removed the criteria that a person "recognises the fear is unreasonable or excessive", noting that people often overestimate the danger involved in given situations, leaving the evaluation of "whether the fear or anxiety is excessive or out of proportion is made by the clinician" (2013a, p. 189).

This differs again from DSM-IV in which the clinician is advised to "review a list of social and performance situations *with* the individual" (1994, p. 413; *emphasis added*). With this particular change, there are inherent risks concerning the erosion of the patient's role and agency in the diagnostic process. Hackmann *et al.* (2019) argue that collaboration between patient and physician in the diagnostic process can help foster a sense of control and empowerment and mitigate the negative consequences, for example, feeling stigmatised, which, in turn, supports engagement with support services and "recovery". Finally, in the most recently published DSM-V-TR (2022a), the diagnostic criteria remain broadly the same (outlined in Table 2.1), but the parenthetical social phobia has been removed entirely, as it "provides no ongoing clinical utility" (APA 2022b, p. 1).

While the DSM "does not take a position about underlying causation" (US Department of Health and Human Services, 1999, p. 44), it has sustained the medicalisation[9] of emotion and behaviour through which various explanatory

Table 2.1 APA Diagnostic Criteria, Social Anxiety Disorder (APA, 2022a, pp. 230–231)

APA Diagnostic Criteria: Social Anxiety Disorder
A. Marked fear or anxiety about one or more social situations in which the individual is exposed to possible scrutiny by others. Examples include social interactions (e.g. having a conversation, meeting unfamiliar people), being observed (e.g. eating or drinking), and performing in front of others (e.g. giving a speech). Note: In children, the anxiety must occur in peer settings and not just during interactions with adults.
B. The individual fears that he or she will act in a way or show anxiety symptoms that will be negatively evaluated (i.e. will be humiliating or embarrassing; will lead to rejection or offend others).
C. The social situations almost always provoke fear or anxiety. Note: In children, fear or anxiety may be expressed by crying, tantrums, freezing, clinging, shrinking, or failing to speak in social situations.
D. The social situations are avoided or endured with intense fear or anxiety.
E. The fear or anxiety is out of proportion to the actual threat posed by the social situation and to the sociocultural context.
F. The fear, anxiety, or avoidance is persistent, typically lasting for six months or more.
G. The fear, anxiety, or avoidance causes clinically significant distress or impairment in social, occupational, or other important areas of functioning.
H. The fear, anxiety, or avoidance is not attributable to the physiological effects of a substance (e.g. a drug of abuse, a medication) or another medical condition.
I. The fear, anxiety, or avoidance is not better explained by the symptoms of another mental disorder, such as panic disorder, body dysmorphic disorder, or autism spectrum disorder.
J. If another medical condition (e.g. Parkinson's disease, obesity, disfigurement from burns or injury) is present, the fear, anxiety, or avoidance is clearly unrelated or excessive.
Specify if: Performance only: If the fear is restricted to speaking or performing in public.

models that intend to account for causative and maintaining factors have been proposed (Aho, 2010). Despite concerns over the "neglected status" of social anxiety, clinical investigations have continued to prioritise neurobiological and cognitive factors that affect social functioning and behaviours. The former promotes the idea that abnormalities in brain structure and function lie at the root of pathological social anxiety disorder (Talati *et al.*, 2013), aspects additionally linked to physiological disturbances (Dewar and Stravynski, 2001). This account also proposes that specific genes may predispose an individual to structural abnormalities and thus, the development of social anxiety disorder (Stravynski 2007), while the latter proposes that dysfunctional beliefs or faulty, irrational or maladaptive cognitions (i.e. thoughts, perceptions and reasoning) results in anxiety and associated behaviours, generating further distress (Clark and Wells, 1995; Stravynski, Bond and Amado, 2004).

The "ontological primacy" (Stravynski 2007, p. 114) of biological and cognitive models loses sight of the social and situational contexts of anxiety – arguably thereby omitting certain aspects of the founding insights from Janet – alongside the layers of meaning and experiences associated with them. In the simplest of terms, there is a loss of what it means and feels like to be anxious in a world shared with others, especially one in which "enterprising characteristics" of competition, autonomy, social comparison and personal responsibility are not only central but elevated as markers of success (Hickinbottom-Brawn, 2013, p. 741). Despite alluding to social, spatial, temporal and indeed embodied aspects at the heart of the anxious experience, the social conditions and contingencies of people's lives are routinely side-lined. The implication is that anxious distress is rendered an individualised condition, operating independently of time and place and devoid of emotional, embodied and social context. Ironically perhaps this version of individuality does not extend to the level of subjective experience, only to its individualised biological underpinnings.

Social underpinnings of social anxiety

Research addressing the social underpinnings of social anxiety has circulated around two main themes. First, by offering sustained criticism of dominant models and providing alternative perspectives. In addition, by framing a critical analysis of the social conditions that enabled social anxiety disorder as a diagnostic category to flourish (Stravynski, 2007; Lane, 2008; Aho, 2010; Hickinbottom-Brawn, 2013) Second, a small body of work has prioritised the social meaning and context of those experiences, how people understand, make sense of and manage social anxiety – and related constructs of embarrassment, shyness and social fears – and how daily life, senses of self and recoveries are lived through and navigated (Scott, 2007; McCarthy, 2014; Boyle, 2019; Yli-Länttä, 2020; Masters, 2021).

Research proposing an *inter*personal model seeks to understand social anxiety as embedded in social roles, norms, communities and practices, indelibly shaped by social institutions and structures (Stravynski, 2014). Stravynski (2007, 2014) takes a critical stance against biological and cognitive models or any characterisation of social phobia as a disease entity caused by defective internal mechanisms. Their alternative interpersonal model proposes that social phobia is "other-orientated, played out in social context" and enacted through "fearful self-protective interpersonal patterns" (2014, p. 7), but there are still some limitations to this approach. While attempting to account for "whole living beings", arguing that both experiences of anxiety and self-protective strategies do not "occur in a vacuum" (Stravynski, 2014, p. xiv), he unfortunately neglects the "intrapersonal dynamics", that is the cognitions and bodily processes, signs and symptoms of distress, arguing that these aspects are too closely associated with and therefore reinforce biological models. Arguably, this omission appeals to his rejection of biological and cognitive models that view "abnormal" cognitions and bodily processes as the "whole problem" – a rejection with which I can greatly sympathise with – but in doing so, he ignores the personal and social consequences of such emotional, embodied and affective events, aspects which I will purposefully pick up and revisit throughout the remainder of this book. Recognition of such embodied responses to social threats, fears and environments are vital as they serve as "protective functions and demonstrate human capacity for meaning-making and agency" (Johnstone and Boyle, M. 2020, p. 1), which makes it imperative that they are accounted for and contextualised within a person's lived experience. Finally, his work is not necessarily critical of diagnostic classifications and often falls back on them, particularly where it seeks to further deepen the medicalisation of anxious distress, proposing that social phobia should in fact sit "somewhere on the spectrum between anxiety disorders and personality disorders" (Stravynski, 2007, p. 138).

A highly pertinent contribution relevant to my own orientation is Scott's critical works on the sociologies of shyness (Scott, 2004, 2005, 2006, 2007). The overriding critique offered by this work concerns the medicalisation of shy identities through diagnostic frameworks of social anxiety disorder and avoidant personality disorder. Scott argues that shyness is both a "personal experience and a social performance" (Scott, 2004, p. 128) and that shy identities, which stand in opposition to the assertive, entrepreneurial and competitive self that is idealised in contemporary Western societies, have been reframed through moralising discourses as a personal failing, deviant behaviour and indicative of apparent "otherness" – ultimately, the very features that Hickinbottom-Brawn (2013) argues rendered shyness susceptible to pathologisation in the first instance. Crucially, Scott attends to the lived experience of shyness and the interactional contexts within which it emerges, drawing attention to how shyness, unfolding in social interactions with others, calls into question "social competence", shaping self-perceptions as well as the wider "norms and values that define what is 'unacceptable' conduct and inform the social reaction to them" (Scott, 2004, p. 132). Elsewhere, McCarthy examines personal recovery journeys of people experiencing "problematic social anxiety", arguing that, by entering the mental health system, receiving a diagnosis and particular therapeutic treatments, people are given a "template for understanding and responding to their emotional distress" (2004, p. 62), which is absorbed, accepted and resisted in various ways and to varying degrees (Chapter 5). Exploring young people's social fears, Yli-Länttä (2020) highlights that "fears were situational and dependent on social changes", adding that meanings derived from them were shaped by the context of the situation and influenced by the relations to other people involved. Finally, Masters (2021) examines how traditional gender roles and norms of femininity impact experiences of social anxiety, arguing that "female socialisation fosters feelings of inadequacy in tandem with creating [a sense of] separateness from the self" (Masters, 2021, p. 310), which are easily co-opted and pathologised by diagnostic systems.

Concluding remarks

Over the course of its 120-year history, there has been a slow but steady erosion of the social and spatial dynamics that underpin the experience of social anxiety. The social and interior worlds, indeed suffering, of the individual, "once core province[s]" (Lie and Greene, 2021, p. 338) of mental healthcare, have been side-lined in favour of increasingly "brain-based" explanations. The "biologisation" of mental illness and increasing "atomisation" of the individual are "flooding zones of human affect that are not pathological, but normal" (Sadowsky, 2021, p. 492) responses to adverse, even traumatic, life circumstances and events. Lost in these reductive approaches is not only the variety of ways social threats and adversities are experienced and expressed over the course of daily life but also the identities, meanings and strategies that are shaped by them. The offerings of sociological accounts are indeed more reflective of the social and cultural contexts that people with social anxiety find themselves having to navigate but we should caution approaches that either reinforce or fall back into unhelpful diagnostic classifications or view social anxiety as wholly continuous with shyness or embarrassment, albeit these may be aspects of some people's experiences. This is a complicated tension, one that requires perhaps having a modicum of ambivalence, as articulated by Callard (2014), towards psychiatric diagnosis but also upholding the very real, intense and disruptive impact of social anxiety on those who live with – sometimes suffering and enduring, but also managing and resisting – it and its consequences.

Notes

1 This brief undertaking of the history of social anxiety takes cues from far more detailed and in-depth explorations and examinations of the development of social anxiety disorder, specifically work by Lloyd (2006), Stravynski (2007, 2008), Lane (2008) and Hickinbottom-Brawn (2013), all of which offer critical and detailed analyses of the history, creation and emergence of social phobia/social anxiety disorder as a diagnostic category.
2 The APA's DSM is primarily used in the USA for psychiatric diagnosis whereas, in the UK and elsewhere, the World Health Organisation's International Classification

of Diseases, currently in its 11th revision (World Health Organisation, 2022) is used. However, I am referencing the former here because the DSM is instrumental in influencing study design and inclusion/exclusion criteria for research, and in constructions of pathology and normalcy, which subsequently shape how disorders are conceptualised, understood and utilised (Halpin, 2016).

3 I am conscious that I am leaving out a much broader history of the concept of anxiety here. Considered central to the human condition, it is a concept that has found great utility in philosophy, theology, medicine, art, literature, psychology, psychiatry, psychoanalysis and social studies across cultures and eras. There is simply not space to cover this here, and extensive works have already been published (Bergo, 2020; Crocq, 2015; Horwitz, 2013; Salecl, 2004).

4 The works of Pierre Janet were written and published in French and have not been translated into English.

5 I am grateful to Dr. Nathalie Prevost for checking the French-to-English translations throughout this chapter.

6 Lloyd notes that while Janet is credited "as a founder of the diagnostic category" (2006, p. 33) in French psychiatry, he is not mentioned in the early English language clinical engagements with the disorder. However, later histories of the disorder have drawn attention to his role and contribution (Stravynski, 2007; Lane, 2008), and arguably, his early insights foreshadow my own explicitly social and spatial concerns.

7 The extent to which the "biologisation" and medicalisation of mental illness has "led to an alleviation, or even a neutralization, of the negative response it inspires" (Guimón and Fischer, 1999, p. viii) is contested. There is not space to cover these arguments here (see: Hinshaw, 2009; Kvaale, Haslam and Gottdiener, 2013).

8 The Task Force oversees the entirety of the DSM project, including the various working groups, for example, the Anxiety Disorders Work Group.

9 To clarify some terms here: "medicalisation" and "pathologisation" are closely linked to each other and often used interchangeably but there are distinctions to be made. Broadly, the former refers to the relocating of distress, inclusive of thoughts, feelings and behaviours, in the individual's psychology or physiology. The latter is implemented in relation to the reconfiguration of behaviours that lie "outside the norms" of "civil" society as "deviant", leading to an unnecessary "medicalisation" of certain aspects of human life (see: Liebert, 2014).

References

Aho, K. (2010) 'The psychopathology of American shyness: A hermeneutic reading', *Journal for the Theory of Social Behaviour*, 40(2), pp. 190–206.

American Psychiatric Association (1980) *Diagnostic and Statistical Manual of Mental Disorders*. 3rd Edition. Washington, DC: American Psychiatric Association.

American Psychiatric Association (1987) *Diagnostic and Statistical Manual of Mental Disorders*. Third Edition, Revised. Washington, DC: American Psychiatric Association.

American Psychiatric Association (1994) *Diagnostic and Statistical Manual of Mental Disorders*. 4th Edition. Washington, DC: American Psychiatric Association.

American Psychiatric Association (2013a) *Diagnostic and Statistical Manual of Mental Disorders*. 5th Edition. Washington, DC: American Psychiatric Association. https://doi.org/10.1176/appi.books.9780890425596

American Psychiatric Association (2013b) 'DSM-V development: Social anxiety disorder fact sheet.' 3b). DSM-V development: Social anxiety disorder fact sheet. (Accessed: 24 April 2023).

American Psychiatric Association (2022a) *Diagnostic and Statistical Manual of Mental Disorders*. 5th Edition, Text Revision. Washington, DC: American Psychiatric Association. https://doi.org/10.1176/appi.books.9780890425787

American Psychiatric Association (2022b) *Social Anxiety Disorder*. Communications. American Psychiatric Association. https://www.psychiatry.org/getmedia/18acfc35-bf15-4c61-b1c8-9a05b0fafc1f/APA-DSM5TR-SocialAnxietyDisorder.pdf (Accessed: 11 September 2023).

Bergo, B. (2020) *Anxiety: A Philosophical History*. Oxford University Press.

Berrios, G. (1999) Anxiety Disorders: A Conceptual History, *Journal of Affective Disorders*, 56(2–3), pp 83–94.

Boyle, L. (2019) 'The (un)habitual geographies of Social Anxiety Disorder', *Social Science & Medicine*, 231, pp. 31–37. https://doi.org/10.1016/j.socscimed.2018.03.002

Callard, F. (2014) 'Psychiatric diagnosis: the indispensability of ambivalence', *Journal of Medical Ethics*, 40(8), pp. 526–530. https://doi.org/10.1136/medethics-2013-101763

Clark, D.M. and Wells, A. (1995) 'A cognitive model of social phobia', in R.G. Heimberg (ed.) *Social Phobia: Diagnosis, Assessment, and Treatment*. Guilford Press, pp. 69–93.

Crocq, M.-A. (2015) 'A history of anxiety: from Hippocrates to DSM', *Dialogues in Clinical Neuroscience*, 17(3), pp. 319–325.

Dewar, K.M. and Stravynski, A. (2001) 'The quest for biological correlates of social phobia: an interim assessment', *Acta Psychiatrica Scandinavica*, 103(4), pp. 244–251. https://doi.org/10.1034/j.1600-0447.2001.00090.x

Dixon, J.J., Monchaux, C. De and Sandler, J. (1957) 'Patterns of anxiety: An analysis of social anxieties*', *British Journal of Medical Psychology*, 30(2), pp. 107–112. https://doi.org/10.1111/j.2044-8341.1957.tb01951.x

Guimón, J. and Fischer, W. (1999) *The Image of Madness: The Public Facing Mental Illness and Psychiatric Treatment*. Karger Medical and Scientific Publishers.

Hackmann, C. et al. (2019) 'Collaborative diagnosis between clinician and patient: why to do it and what to consider', *BJPsych Advances*, 25(4), pp. 214–222. https://doi.org/10.1192/bja.2019.6

Halpin, M. (2016) 'The DSM and professional practice: Research, clinical, and institutional perspectives', *Journal of Health and Social Behavior*, 57(2), pp. 153–167. https://doi.org/10.1177/0022146516645637

Hickinbottom-Brawn, S. (2013) 'Brand "you": The emergence of social anxiety disorder in the age of enterprise', *Theory & Psychology*, 23(6), pp. 732–751. https://doi.org/10.1177/0959354313500579

Hinshaw, S.P. (2009) *The Mark of Shame: Stigma of Mental Illness and an Agenda for Change*. Oxford University Press.

Horwitz, A.V. (2013) *Anxiety: A Short History*. Johns Hopkins University Press. Available at: https://doi.org/10.1353/book.26766

Hummelen, B. et al. (2007) 'The relationship between avoidant personality disorder and social phobia', *Comprehensive Psychiatry*, 48(4), pp. 348–356. https://doi.org/10.1016/j.comppsych.2007.03.004

Huppert, J.D. et al. (2008) 'Generalized social anxiety disorder and avoidant personality disorder: structural analysis and treatment outcome', *Depression and Anxiety*, 25(5), pp. 441–448. https://doi.org/10.1002/da.20349

Janet, P. (1903) *Les obsessions et la psychasthénie*. Edited by F. Alcan. Travaux du Laboratoire de Psychologie de la Clinique à la Salpêtrière (Troisième Série).

Johnstone, L. and Boyle, M. (2020) *The power threat meaning framework: towards the identification of patterns in emotional distress, unusual experiences and troubled or troubling behaviour, as an alternative to functional psychiatric diagnosis.*

Kato, T.A., Kanba, S. and Teo, A.R. (2018) 'Hikikomori: experience in Japan and international relevance', *World Psychiatry*, 17(1), pp. 105–106. https://doi.org/10.1002/wps.20497

Kirmayer, L.J. and Pedersen, D. (2014) 'Toward a new architecture for global mental health', *Transcultural Psychiatry*, 51(6), pp. 759–776. https://doi.org/10.1177/1363461514557202

Kvaale, E.P., Haslam, N. and Gottdiener, W.H. (2013) 'The "side effects" of medicalization: A meta-analytic review of how biogenetic explanations affect stigma', *Clinical Psychology Review*, 33(6), pp. 782–794. https://doi.org/10.1016/j.cpr.2013.06.002

Lane, C. (2008) *Shyness: How Normal Behavior Became a Sickness.* Yale University Press.

Lane, C. (2022) *Robert Spitzer on DSM-III: A Recently Recovered Interview, Mad In America.* https://www.madinamerica.com/2022/02/robert-spitzer-dsm/ (Accessed: 20 April 2023).

Lie, A.K. and Greene, J. (2021) 'Introduction to special issue: Psychiatry as social medicine', *Culture, Medicine, and Psychiatry*, 45(3), pp. 333–342. https://doi.org/10.1007/s11013-021-09740-7

Liebert, R. (2014) 'Pathologization', in T. Teo (ed.) *Encyclopedia of Critical Psychology.* Springer, pp. 1327–1333. https://doi.org/10.1007/978-1-4614-5583-7_572

Liebowitz, M.R. (2010) 'The emergence of social anxiety disorder as a major medical condition', in F. Schneier et al. (eds) *Anxiety Disorders: Theory, Research and Clinical Perspectives.* Cambridge University Press, pp. 40–49. https://doi.org/10.1017/CBO9780511777578.006

Liebowitz, M.R. et al. (1985) 'Social phobia. Review of a neglected anxiety disorder', *Archives of General Psychiatry*, 42(7), pp. 729–736. https://doi.org/10.1001/archpsyc.1985.01790300097013

Lloyd, S. (2006) *An Anxious Society: The French Importation of Social Phobia and the Appearance of a New Model of the Self.* McGill University. https://escholarship.mcgill.ca/concern/theses/wp988q019 (Accessed: 10 September 2023).

Marks, I.M. and Gelder, M.G. (1966) 'Different ages of onset in varieties of phobia', *American Journal of Psychiatry*, 123(2), pp. 218–221. https://doi.org/10.1176/ajp.123.2.218

Marks, I.M. (1969) *Fears and Phobias.* London: Academic Press.

Masters, K. (2021) *Putting the 'Social' in 'Social Anxiety Disorder': Exploring Women's Experiences from a Feminist and Anti-Psychiatry Perspective.* Unpublished PhD Thesis. University of Birmingham.

Mayes, R. and Horwitz, A.V. (2005) 'DSM-III and the revolution in the classification of mental illness', *Journal of the History of the Behavioral Sciences*, 41(3), pp. 249–267. https://doi.org/10.1002/jhbs.20103

McCarthy, C. (2014) *Social Anxiety: Personal Narratives on Journeys to Recovery.* Unpublished PhD Thesis. University of East London.

Sadowsky, J. (2021) 'Before and after prozac: Psychiatry as medicine, and the historiography of depression', *Culture, Medicine, and Psychiatry*, 45(3), pp. 479–502. https://doi.org/10.1007/s11013-021-09729-2

Salecl, R. (2004) *On Anxiety.* Routledge. http://archive.org/details/onanxiety0000sale (Accessed: 8 September 2023).

Scott, S. (2004) 'The shell, the stranger and the competent other: Towards a sociology of shyness', *Sociology*, 38(1), pp. 121–137. https://doi.org/10.1177/0038038504039364

Scott, S. (2005) 'The red, shaking fool: Dramaturgical dilemmas in shyness', *Symbolic Interaction*, 28(1), pp. 91–110. https://doi.org/10.1525/si.2005.28.1.91

Scott, S. (2006) 'The medicalisation of shyness: from social misfits to social fitness', *Sociology of Health & Illness*, 28(2), pp. 133–153. https://doi.org/10.1111/j.1467-9566.2006.00485.x

Scott, S. (2007) *Shyness and Society*. Palgrave Macmillan UK. https://doi.org/10.1057/9780230801325_7

Stravynski, A. (2007) *Fearing Others: The Nature and Treatment of Social Phobia*. Cambridge University Press.

Stravynski, A. (2014) *Social Phobia: An Interpersonal Approach*. Cambridge University Press.

Stravynski, A., Bond, S. and Amado, D. (2004) 'Cognitive causes of social phobia: A critical appraisal', *Clinical Psychology Review*, 24(4), pp. 421–440. https://doi.org/10.1016/j.cpr.2004.01.006

Talati, A. et al. (2013) 'Grey matter abnormalities in social anxiety disorder: Primary, replication, and specificity studies', *Biological Psychiatry*, 73(1), p. 75. https://doi.org/10.1016/j.biopsych.2012.05.022

Tanaka-Matsumi, J. (1979) 'Taijin Kyofusho: Diagnostic and cultural issues in Japanese psychiatry', *Culture, Medicine and Psychiatry*, 3(3), pp. 231–245. https://doi.org/10.1007/BF00114612

Tyrer, P. (2018) 'Against the stream: Generalised anxiety disorder (GAD) – A redundant diagnosis', *BJPsych Bulletin*, 42(2), pp. 69–71. https://doi.org/10.1192/bjb.2017.12

US Department of Health and Human Services (1999) *Mental Health: A Report of the Surgeon General*. MD; US: Department of Health and Human Services, Substance Abuse and Mental Health Services Administration, Center for Mental Health Services, National Institutes of Health, National Institute of Mental Health. https://profiles.nlm.nih.gov/spotlight/nn/catalog/nlm:nlmuid-101584932X120-doc (Accessed: 11 September 2023).

Valsiner, J. and van der Veer, R. (2000) *The Social Mind: Construction of the Idea*. Cambridge University Press. http://archive.org/details/socialmindconstr0000vals_c4h4 (Accessed: 10 September 2023).

Widiger, T.A. (1992) 'Generalized social phobia versus avoidant personality disorder: a commentary on three studies', *Journal of Abnormal Psychology*, 101(2), pp. 340–343. https://doi.org/10.1037//0021-843x.101.2.340

World Health Organisation (2022) *The ICD-11 Classification of Mental and Behavioural Disorders: Diagnostic Criteria for Research*. 11th Edition. World Health Organisation.

Yli-Länttä, H. (2020) 'Young people's experiences of social fears', *International Journal of Adolescence and Youth*, 25(1), pp. 1022–1035. https://doi.org/10.1080/0267384 3.2020.1828110

3 Situating social anxiety

Introduction

This chapter situates social anxiety within the geographies of health, illness and wellbeing. Drawing conceptually from humanistic and posthuman concerns that have enriched geographical understandings of health, the conceptual underpinnings for this research are outlined. Broadly, it pivots on three interrelated conceptual points: spatialities, temporalities and embodiments, and related themes therein. Each aspect will emerge, be expanded upon, and be contextualised in varying moves, degrees and interactions throughout the empirically based chapters that follow. Collectively, they should be regarded as a "sensitising framework" through which the everyday contingencies and complexities of the anxious experience can be recognised, understood and communicated.

Geographies of health and wellbeing

At the heart of this book is a concern with the phenomenological potentials of new configurations of humanism (Simonsen, 2013) and post-humanism (Andrews, 2019) for cultivating a geographical understanding of social anxiety and the mundane and not-so-mundane contexts and contingencies through which it is experienced. As Philo (2007, p. 89) notes, humanism and post-humanism(s) – together with their associated concerns with, respectively, the representational and non-representational; reflective and pre-reflective; personal and pre-personal; thought and practice; emotion and affect; discourse and materiality, – "cannot but sit uneasily" alongside one another. So, before attending to the various ways in which these approaches are conceptualised and mobilised throughout this book, it feels necessary to address briefly the conflicting, often polarised, positions of humanistic and post-humanistic thought within the geographies of health (and the discipline, more broadly) and how this research is positioned in relation to this "conflict".

It has been 30 years since Kearns (1993) proposed a "post-medical geography" that considers the wider links between health and place. The idea being that an approach to medical geography "released from the shadow of medicine"

DOI: 10.4324/9781003206880-3

(Kearns and Gesler, 1998, p. 5) and attentive to the situated and experiential, rather than biomedical, could engage more relational and holistic accounts of health, illness and wellbeing by acknowledging the social dimensions through which experience is constructed and mediated. *Place* became the key orientating concept around which to re-engage the rich and complex ways whereby people engage with, understand and construct the world around them, paying particular attention to experiential aspects alongside the processes of agency and meaning-making inherent in negotiating health and care. These early interventions are captured in geographical engagements with the therapeutic and healing capacities of physical, symbolic and social environments (Gesler, 1992; Williams, 2007) and at the heart of geographies of ageing, care and responsibility (Rowles, 2000; Conradson, 2003). Retaining these early humanistic sentiments concerned with the experiential dimensions of life but responding to its inherent limitations with "renewed recognition of diversity and difference" (Kearns, 1993, p. 145), critical geographies re-engaged with health at the intersections of race, class, gender and sexuality (Kearns, 1995; Wilton, 1996; Moss, 1997; Del Casino Jr, 2007). More recently, geographical approaches have been "enlivened" by posthuman concerns for "de-centring" the human being as the focus of social inquiry, accenting affective, vital and more-than-human events and relations – and associated assemblages of human and non-human forces – at play in the process and practice of health and wellbeing (Atkinson, 2013; Duff, 2016; Andrews, 2018).

While finding utility in the posthuman offerings of non-representational approaches to affect, practice, materiality and their relational embodiments, this project is not a "non-representational" one in that it centres more phenomenological and humanistic concerns with lived experience, (inter)subjectivity, agency, identity, meaning-making and senses of belonging and place.[1] It is also attentive to the "speaking subject" (i.e. reliant on typed and spoken words through online questionnaire and interview techniques) (Chapter 1) with the intent "to engage the registers of affect, feeling […] and other forms of bodily knowing" (Blackman and Venn, 2010, p. 18), specifically because these voices are all too often overlooked and dismissed in research *about* them. However, this concern for the "*speakable* qualities and 'storyable' characteristics" (Laurier and Philo, 2006, 358; *original italics*) of the anxious experience is coupled with a recognition of their limitations – in that what is remembered, omitted, written or spoken, may not correspond to actual experience or reality; may remain inaccessible to consciousness, be misrepresented, enacted automatically or voluntarily; and can, and often does, escape or exceed linguistic representation – but also nonetheless accepts that even failures and distortions of representation, especially those that representative of mental and emotional distress, are deeply entangled with and dependent on perceptions and past experiences (De Timary, et al. 2011) (Chapter 4). In the psychoanalytic context, for example, part of the analysts role is aiding the patient in rediscovering the links between representation and matters of affect, movement or practice (De Timary et al. 2011). While it is not the intention of this research to clarify all these links nor get to the "root cause" of the anxious experience, it proceeds from two positions: first, the representations of experiences offered in this research are significant to the speaker and as such they are embodied, complex, and even contradictory; second, they are not conceived as solely "representative" of a person's inner world, but rather reflect a wider "community of content" (De Timary, et al. 2011), imbued not only with personal experience but also inflected by wider mediating structures, social conventions, common "senses", and complex acts of meaning-making. From this juncture, I seek a "dialogue" between the binary oppositions outlined above (Philo, 2007), and I envision an approach more akin to what Simonsen conceives of as "the phenomenological travel along the [...] post-humanist lane" (2013, p. 22).

The task here, therefore, is to work *with* representations to aid an embodied account that stories the anxious body as embedded in, contingent upon and emerges through its interactions with others and the social practices that comprise daily life (Simonsen, 2013). Biomedical knowledge and practice are of course often taken as synonymous with "the body": a body often viewed as a material and machine-like object, divisible and reducible to a collection of isolable physical parts, systems and processes (Marcum, 2005) and atomised "into the smallest of biologically recognised fragments" (Sharp, 2000, p. 309). It is a body depersonalised and decontextualised, removed from the social and cultural milieu, and deanimated, disembodied from selfhood, identity and subjectivity and void of experiences and emotions (Leder, 1992). In response, a geography attentive to the embodiments of health and illness clearly necessitates a "reinterpretation of biology" (Hall, 2000, p. 22), with attention to embodiment proceeding from the reciprocal conditioning that takes place between body and world. Phenomenological approaches in this connection are concerned with the body's "double ontology", approaching "the body as 'body-as-subject', as a seat of feeling, movement, agency and activity; and the 'body-as-object', as felt, observed, and acted upon" (Slatman, 2014, p. 555). The body is understood as having a simultaneous and reciprocal possibility for understanding, making sense of and acting in the world, both reflectively and pre-reflectively, while itself being conditioned by the world (Slatman, 2014). By prioritising the lived body as a site of experience, my work here aims to resituate the body within the social world through interrelated dimensions of embodied meanings, embodied practices and affectivities – aspects that are, in and of themselves, spatially and temporally situated and mediated.

Addressing the intersecting complexities of the anxious experience through a geographical lens, and attending to the omissions in the anxiety research landscape, necessitates attention to the affective, sensorial and corporeal dimensions of experience. More specifically, those affective experiences that are currently quantified and interpreted within biomedical domains as the signs and symptoms of disorder rather than responses to threatening personal and social situations (Johnstone and Boyle, 2020). This juncture, which lends itself to more "localised" conceptualisation of affect that is: "context-specific and situated" (Kidd and MacArthur, 2019, p. 1748); intends to resituate the human subject by paying attention to the discursive and emotive body (Thien, 2005), aligns with approaches that have perhaps been side-lined by the recent furore of posthuman and non-representational attentions, but that are broadly critical of conceptualisations of affect situated *contra* the emotional, the discursive and the cognitive (Thien, 2005; Laurier and Philo, 2006; Tolia-Kelly, 2006; Papoulias and Callard, 2010; Leys, 2011; Wetherell, 2013).

Through this approach, the experience of social anxiety is resituated as a mode of existence, a way of being-in-the-world, that fluctuates, advances and retreats, that resonates through the body and across social space, and emerges in and through affective practices at various spatial and temporal orientations. It is an approach that is sensitive to the co-constitution and mutual entanglements of these different phenomena. This chapter now turns to the conceptual underpinnings that this research builds upon and through which the above discussion and overall experience of social anxiety are navigated: namely, the intertwining capacities of spatialities, temporalities and embodiments.

Spatialities

The geographies explored throughout this section contribute to and build upon relational approaches in the geographies of mental health that prioritise the social and spatial contexts and contingencies shaping the lived experience of mental and emotional distress. Over the last 20 years, research in the geographies of mental health has been broadly concerned with three interrelated threads of inquiry. First, the personal geographies of particular conditions and the spatial manifestations of mental and emotional distress, including agoraphobia and panic (Davidson, 2000; Bankey, 2004; Sánchez-Rodillo Espeso, 2022); bipolar disorder (Chouinard, 2012); obsessive-compulsive disorder (OCD) (Segrott and Doel, 2004); seasonal affective disorder (Bodden *et al.*, 2022); specific phobias (Davidson, 2005); suicide and self-harm (Stevenson, 2016); voice-hearing, visions and unusual beliefs (Parr, 1999; Nieuwenhuis and Knoll, 2021); and mental distress, broadly defined (Tucker, 2010). The second thread of investigation lends itself to the therapeutic and harmful potential of specific places and spaces, including home (Davidson, 2000; Holmes, 2008); workplaces (Evans and Wilton, 2019); supermarkets (Davidson, 2001); community clubhouses (Martin, 2021); self-help groups (Laws, 2009); hospitals (Wood *et al.*, 2015); asylums (Parr, Philo and Burns, 2003); drop-in centres (Parr, 2000); and online spaces (Campbell and Longhurst, 2013). The final thread consists of the everyday practices and mobilities that make up these spaces, including coping strategies (Boyle, 2019); help-seeking (Tucker and Lavis, 2019); recovery work (Laws, 2013); and artistic, creative and therapeutic practices (Parr, 2006, 2007; McGeachan, 2017). This body of research is broadly concerned with people's personal and "experiential worlds" (McGeachan, 2017, p. 4) and the various ways that space and place are constitutive of health and wellbeing. The subjective underpinnings of this work disrupt the reductive and depersonalised frameworks of biomedical models of mental health and help to bring "more sharply into view the faces and voices of people with mental health problems" (Parr, 2008, pp. 11–12). Within this diverse body of inquiry salient themes emerge concerned with how "self-other-world" relations are implicated in and integral to shaping everyday experiences and understandings of anxious distress.

Davidson's work on the geographies of agoraphobia is instructive for considering troubling bodily events that fundamentally interfere with the capacity to lead fulfilling social and spatial lives. Davidson details not only the "difficulties [faced] in traversing social space" but also the "complete breakdown of the boundaries between 'inner' self and 'outer' world" (2000, p. 641). A person's sense of self, security and identity can be fractured along these boundaries between inside-outside. Similarly, attempts to quell distressing and intrusive thoughts (obsessions) through repetitive actions (compulsions) demonstrate how boundaries are actively managed and maintained as a self-protective strategy, often to distressing extents, for example, a fear that certain objects and spaces are contaminated may be alleviated by lengthy cleansing rituals, ordering objects or expelling them from the space altogether (Segrott and Doel, 2004).

Another crucial aspect is the interplay between self and other, and how these interactions and relationships allow "us" to make sense of ourselves, and others, as social beings in different contexts. This can promote or disrupt senses of identity or belonging through processes and practices of recognition and misrecognition, denial and connection, inclusion and exclusion, which may often be bound up in wider systems of policy and power. McGrath et al. (2008) demonstrate the supportive capacity of others, arguing that access to like-minded people in safe online environment can nurture positive social connections for those experiencing anxiety. On the other hand, "dismissive [and] denigrating attitudes" from others about particular fears and phobias may "contribute to the secrecy and stigma surrounding the experience and perception of phobias" (Davidson, 2005, p. 2155). Similarly, Parr et al. examine the complex and ambiguous social and spatial dynamics of inclusion and exclusion experienced by mental health service users in rural localities whereby illness, and specifically people's reactions to it, can "cement or disrupt senses of community embeddedness" (2004, 406).

Finally, various social and physical environments are identified as being simultaneous or ambiguous sources of support and strife at different times and under certain conditions. In contrast to crowded public spaces, home often provides a "secure base" that is "private [and] bounded" and safe from external threats for people with agoraphobia (Holmes, 2008, p. 375), while at the same time then potentially becoming a "trap", hereby associated with negative feelings for those who end up (self-)confined to a domestic setting. Tellingly, in this case what was once a "sanctuary" may end up a "prison", a switch of considerable significance in the life worlds of many with social anxiety (Chapter 6). Drawing on emotional and therapeutic geographies, Wood et al. (2015) demonstrate how emotions and memories can "impinge on one's present therapeutic experience". Parr, Philo and Burns (2003) uncover the "contested meanings" of institutional spaces such as "old" asylum buildings and grounds, highlighting that feelings of community and care often co-exist alongside more fearful geographies of surveillance and isolation. Other therapeutic programmes, spaces and practices can shape people's identities and feelings of "wellness" – such as art programmes or community gardening groups as vehicles to foster social inclusion and sense of belonging (Parr, 2007) or social enterprises and therapeutic workplaces promoting a "sense of belonging tied to socially valued roles" (Evans and Wilton, 2019, p. 80) – but even here the experience can be double-edged, both affirmative for those who thrive on these practice-based sites and alienating for others who may simply wish "to be" rather than to act or work (Philo, Parr and Burns, 2005). Crucially indeed, studies in this vein have been cautious of the "transformative" and "integrative" capacities of such social-welfare projects for typically marginalised and vulnerable people, as they are often defined here in relation to discourses of active and responsible citizenship present in health and social policy objectives.

Temporalities

The experience of health and illness is subject to both objective and subjective conceptualisations of time (Toombs, 1990). The temporal regimes of medical and psychiatric discourse are largely grounded in objective conceptualisations of time that assume measurability and neutrality. This one-directional flow of time, typically syncing with clocks and calendars, frames the course of diagnosis, prognosis and treatment. Particular constructions of illness are also shaped temporally in relation to duration or frequency through terms such as: "chronic", "intermittent", "acute", "persistent" and "remission", in which time is conceived of as "a neutral coordinate that exists independently of other factors" (von Peter, 2010, p. 14). Yet, this objective sense of time plays a powerful role in governing how people understand, live with and manage health and illness, setting the pace of, and trajectories for, "recovery" (where or if, at all, possible) but nonetheless often shaping health behaviours and expectations. Such temporal orderings are evident in the role of prognosis, for determining the timing and staging of illness (Sakellariou, Nissen and Warren, 2021); in vital routine appointments and procedures for kidney dialysis (Vestman et al. 2014) or chemotherapy (Rasmussen and Elverdam, 2007); in the temporalities of organ transplant surgery (Wasson, 2021); in the time-lines and targets set for mental health recovery (McWade, 2015); in drug treatment programmes for addiction (Schlosser, 2018); in the importance of patient history in the treatment of chronic pain, particularly the duration and frequency of pain (Nilsen and Elstad, 2009); the frequency of seizures in epilepsy (Smith, 2012); and the routine management practices required in diabetes (Lucherini, 2020). As Sakellariou et al. (2021, p. 144) note, there is an "expectation that biomedicine provides an indication of what [the] future might look like, how things might develop over time [...] and how people might live and care during that period", and yet how often does biomedicine fail to take into account how time is directly encountered and experienced by patients and service users. The research outlined above overwhelmingly demonstrates and aims to rectify the disparity between the temporal inscriptions of biomedicine, which offers a "discrete snapshot" (Nilsen and Elstad, 2009, p. 52) of ongoing life-shaping events. Moreover, such inscriptions may be restrictive, disruptive, disorienting, tedious or incompatible with the commitments, responsibilities and indeed realities of everyday life. This research also shows in a variety of ways how biomedical temporalities and practices shape not only the expectations and experiences of health, illness and treatment, but bodies and subjectivities too, cutting off and de-potentialising certain other ways of being with unwellness.

As Andrews (2021) notes, explicit engagements with time and temporality in health geography are limited (for exceptions, see: Driedger, et al., 2004; McQuoid, et al. 2017; Lucherini, 2020), compared to the temporally-orientated work in the sociologies of health and illness, particularly in chronic illness studies (Toombs, 1990; Jowsey, 2016). However, one does not need to look far to see complex temporalities implicated in the lives and subjectivities across a range of health and health-related experiences that have been the focus of geographical inquiry (Andrews, 2021). Andrews (2021) demarcates the temporal ambitions of such geographical research along two threads of inquiry highly relevant to the present research. The first concerns the subjective experience in and of time, what Andrews terms "knowing time". Predominantly framed by phenomenological and humanistic perspectives, these approaches aim to provide greater insights into the "life worlds" of illness. These comprise the lived temporalities of "clock time", synchronisation with others and environments and the experiential flow of past, present and future. The second, underpinned by non-representational approaches, accounts for how time is sensed and created, it is "not concerned with representations of time" but with "what is 'taking-place' right now", defined as the "event", involving both the "physical attributes and embodied experiences" of space and time (Andrews, 2021, p. 6). Intertwined with issues of embodiment discussed in the next section, non-representational approaches are concerned with "performed and felt timings" rather than with the "subjects' feelings about time"(Andrews, 2021, p. 19): that is, the rhythms, practices and mobilities such as those evident in therapeutic practices and holistic routines (Lea, Cadman and Philo, 2015; Boyd, 2017).

The implicit and explicit engagements with time and temporalities across the relevant disciplines can be broadly summarised by the following interrelated threads: restrictive and disruptive temporalities; and layered temporalities. Each captures subjective and nuanced dimensions of health and illness, and the processes and practices that shape individual experiences and personal geographies.

Restrictive and disruptive temporalities

Research in this vein has focused primarily on specific conditions and experiences of illness centred on the duration, stages and events of embodied illness and the implications arising for socio-spatial relations and senses of self. Driedger et al. (2004) draw attention to the temporality of everyday life for people diagnosed with Multiple Sclerosis (MS), assessing how they engage in the process of disablement either through gradual progression over time or through relapsing-remitting cycles of the condition. This cyclical experience is also evident in the seasonal patterns of depression, or "seasonal affective disorder", in which reduced light and lower energy experienced in the winter months "make everyday activities more difficult causing people to feel 'stuck' or 'left behind'" (Bodden *et al.*, 2022, p. 28). The flow of time can often be punctuated by embodied "events", one extreme example being epilepsy, where Smith (2012) notes how seizure frequency (and their relative unpredictability) disrupt the temporal experiences of everyday life for people with epilepsy. The "event" of the seizure is temporally disruptive in and of itself, in that "time stands still" and the "flow" of daily life is punctured by disorientating absences in time. Such disruptions often result in an inability to plan lives (on shorter or longer horizons) marking a further, ongoing form of temporal disruption for people with epilepsy.

Across a range of health experiences, the temporal logics of healing, management or recovery – of "living well" – entail synchronising the routines and rhythms of everyday life with specific treatment and behavioural regimes (Benton *et al.*, 2017) (Chapter 8). Assessing the temporalities of healthcare interventions, Gibson et al. (2022, p. 1162) highlight how the roles of responsibilities of everyday life can often "conflict with the linearity of intervention time", making it impossible to attend appointments and exacerbating existing conditions (Chapter 5). Such temporal logics therefore dictate what support and recovery looks like: for example, while making time for and engaging with specific prescriptions (pharmaceutical, social or otherwise) supposedly demonstrates a commitment to one's "recovery", the lack of specific provisions and therapeutic interventions can often leave individuals without the necessary "continuity and coordination of care" (Jowsey *et al.*, 2016, p. 854). Similarly, Lucherini (2020, p. 7) highlights the social and emotional burden of living with diabetes in which strict routines and self-management practices often serve as a "grinding and constant reminder of the lack of spontaneity and serendipity" afforded to those managing such a chronic illness.

Layered temporalities

The second temporal focus concerns "layered temporalities". Conceptually orientated around considerations of past, present and future, it captures the complexity of time and the extent to which experiences of health, illness and health-related behaviours constitute a disruption in the temporal continuity of life. While chronologically isolable in linear perspectives of time, past, present and future when viewed through the lens of subjectively lived time is more than a simple succession of "what has been", "what is" and "what has yet-to-come". Rather, they are indissolubly interwoven into the fabric of experienced time

(Wyllie, 2005). Present experience is not only shaped by past experiences and driven by/towards anticipated futures but also retroactively shapes and colours past experiences and memories. Past, present and future events can be conceptualised as "existential coordinates" that are integral to grounding and shaping a person's sense of who they are, their experiences and their behaviours (Orona, 1990) (Chapter 4). They are also altering events that "re-order the individual's understanding of [their] past and future, and of [their] identity" (Orona, 1990, p. 1253). With past-orientated concerns, there may be a sense of longing for one's past self or grieving lost parts of one's identity (Charmaz, 1983). Illness experiences, coupled with the requirements of care, impact social roles, livelihoods, resources and activities that are integral for people discerning "who they are" in the world (Fang *et al.*, 2023). This can undermine previously held beliefs and explanations about the self, resulting in feelings of alienation from one's self and body. Equally, there are many future uncertainties related to how life will unfold or be constrained or disrupted by illness, and as a result hoped for and imagined futures "may have to be radically altered or shelved permanently" (Kelly, 2010, p. 16).

Particularly with experiences related to mental and emotional distress, trauma and addiction, there is a disruption, distortion or even discontinuity in the temporal character of past-present-future. Where the past forcefully re-enters the present, as is experienced in PTSD (post-traumatic stress disorder), the temporal experience is repeatedly disrupted through a persistent and recurring "invasion" of negative past memories or "flashbacks". Rather than re-remembering, there is an embodied and traumatic re-living of events which, coupled with dissociation, amounts to "losing time and [...] a coherent sense of self" (Mezzalira, 2022). Similar temporal dimensions and embodied affectivities are unpacked in Chapter 4.

Embodiments

The third conceptual pin concerns the embodiments of health and illness and intends to capture, on the one hand, the profound extent to which social forces (inclusive of social norms, values, expectations, discourses) are part of our daily activities and experiences ("embodied meanings") and, on the other, how the enactment of these meanings shapes our thinking, feeling and acting across different social situations and contexts ("embodied practices"). Attention to the former, in particular, does not intend to "subordinate" the lived experience of the body to "wider" influences, but rather, is a (perhaps ambitious) attempt to attend to "both bodily and social influences together as constituents (but not determinants) of subjectivity and experience" (Cromby, 2014). In the context of social anxiety, embodiment proceeds from an internalised and quantifiable understanding in which the connection to self and others is "flawed" (Varlet *et al.*, 2014). Particularly relevant here (and I would argue, to our understandings of mental health more broadly) is how a person embodies such influences from the outside, in, for example, how one works with and, more importantly, *resists* various social processes and influences, whether that be the process of diagnosis, the medicalisation of their distress and their engagement with practices of recovery (Chapter 5) or in the expectations of motherhood (Chapter 6).

Embodied meaning

There is burgeoning literature theorising "the intersections of bodies, knowledge and power" (Parr, 2002a) in the experience of health and illness, particularly addressing the intricate relationship between oppressive societal systems (such as neoliberalism, patriarchy, racism, ableism) and a diverse array of discourses (including social, cultural, medical, popular narratives). This body of literature scrutinises the multifaceted and intersecting roles played by these systems and discourses, which can act as causative, aggravating or sustaining factors in shaping not only health and illness but also experiences of being in and navigating through the world (Brijnath and Antoniades, 2016; Burke, 2006; Laketa and Côte, 2023; Parr, 2002b). Thus, "embodied meanings" attend to how social discourses, narratives and values may be reflected within habituated practices and behaviours and how bodies are "discursively and practically produced and maintained" (Mehta and Bondi, 1999, p. 69). Psychiatric and psychological discourses are illustrative examples of how powerful discourses are not only embedded in, but implicit in shaping, everyday being. For example, Burke (2006) addresses the connections that feminist scholarship has drawn between anorexia and the influence of patriarchal systems and mass media, teasing out how these systems reinforce gender norms and contribute to the propagation of idealised images of femininity. Laketa and Côte (2023) emphasise the connections between academic burnout and the neoliberalisation of academic institutions, assessing the impact of deteriorating labour conditions on everyday embodiments in the workplace. They argue that rather than individual pathology, burnout is deeply rooted in the social and economic conditions created by neoliberal policies that are resulting in increased workloads, job insecurity, uncertain prospects and competition for jobs and grants. Chapter 5 provides some insights into similar employment struggles for the socially anxious.

Parr (2002b) examines how medical knowledge is variously embodied. First, through the increasing reach of medical knowledges and technologies into daily life through the internet, subsequently shaping how the body is understood, evaluated, surveyed and managed; and second, by highlighting how medical knowledges are absorbed and contested in online forums used by people with MS to help them make sense of their diagnosis while also resisting the medicalisation of their changing bodies (often forum users end up favouring the shared and subjective knowledges of MS communities, "experts" in their own conditions). Others have assessed how neoliberal agendas are embedded in current mental healthcare (and related policy), particularly in relation to the promotion of individual responsibility and autonomy, often with emphasis on self-management. Such narratives encourage patients to take charge of their own care, reducing reliance on state-funded or community support services and fostering market-oriented approaches where individuals are expected to make self-directed choices about their treatment and, as a result, bear more of the financial and personal burden for their care. In the context of depression, Brijnath and Antoniades (2016) address tensions arising between how self-management of illness is promoted and the actual behaviours and strategies that individuals employ when attempting to manage their illness independently. Specifically, these authors address how neoliberal logics are "absorbed and enacted", by patients (Brijnath and Antoniades, 2016, p. 6). They argue that the neoliberal patient's "imperative to self-manage" can have detrimental consequences for overall health and wellbeing since to be "successfully self-managing also meant disengagement [from] health services, self-medication and self-labour" (Brijnath and Antoniades, 2016). Thus, failure to embody self-managing effectively so as to achieve "recovery" can be indicative of individual effort or lack therefore, and hence risk – as discussed already – an emphasis on embodying personal, moral and practical shortcomings.

Embodied practices

Embodied practices are generally concerned with the experiences and *doings* that constitute healthy bodies and therapeutic places (Evans, 2018). Scholarship has highlighted the various ways in which people find health and wellbeing in the teeth of, or in some cases ways of living *through*, adverse health experiences (Power *et al.*, 2019), whether this be through the "therapeutic assemblages" of walking, talking and place (Ireland *et al.*, 2019) or the personal, spatial and temporal "modulations" that enable and curtail recovery from mental illness (Duff, 2016). For those who have experienced a radical disconnection between self and body, embodied physical movements and practice have been engaged as therapeutic tools to renegotiate the relationship with the body, as in the practice of yoga for those living with anorexia nervosa (Lucas, 2022); or in the integrative practices of dance movement psychotherapy for those experiencing voice-hearing and dissociation in psychosis (Coaten, 2022).

Embodiment is almost always conceived (albeit critically) through hopeful and transformative potentials. Yet, there are a number of embodied practices typically conceived as detrimental to health, or often selfish, taboo and unspeakable, isolated in time and place. These include self-medication, drug use, self-harm and suicide, which have been reconceived through a geographical imagination as thoroughly embedded and emplaced acts through which people attempt to adapt to, cope with, respond to, find relief in or be free from, immense personal, emotional and social suffering. Given that people with social anxiety often wait over a decade before seeking medical and/or therapeutic support, self-management strategies, some more detrimental than others to overall health and wellbeing, are regularly engaged into cope with and manage recurring, persistent and fluctuating anxieties (Chapter 8). Stevenson (2016, p. 200), exploring suicidal feelings and attempted suicide, rejects dominant perspectives on suicide as a final, "private and individualised act", arguing instead that suicide is better conceived of as relational "journey", a "complex [and] fragmented set of events unfolding over time", imbued with meaning, marked by feelings of belonging and alienation, and thoroughly embodied in ordinary places. Simopoulou and Chandler (2020) explore self-harming practices as both a personally significant act and an attempt at self-care. They trouble notions that typically conceive of self-harm as either "attention seeking" or a "violent attack" in which "the body is portrayed as vandalised and almost deserted" (2020, p. 114); rather, it is a means of relating to and recognising a body variously experienced as numb, "unfeeling", empty or dead. The body is shaped through the repetition of the act, re-experienced as alive and real, even if offering only a temporary and fleeting release; and through the permanence of bodily scars that marks the experience and the body as "valid concrete and seen" (2020, p. 117).

Concluding remarks

In summary, I would propose that standard understandings of social anxiety are dominated by individualistic accounts, removed from the personal and social contexts that provoke, give meaning to and sustain anxious distress. As a corrective to these approaches, the chapters that follow provide a social account, grounded in notions of spatiality, temporality and embodied subjectivity, and constituted through the interactions of feeling, perception, practice and discourse. Throughout, social anxiety is re-conceptualised as a social and spatial phenomenon, co-constituted and contingent upon relational, social and spatial influences. Examining the social and situated aspects of social anxiety draws attention not only to the content and context of social anxiety, but enables a deeper understanding of the many overlapping contours of anxious distress, including its restrictive and disruptive capacity, the various ways it is enacted and sustained; its association with avoidance, withdrawal and isolation; the feelings of uncertainty, disconnection and detachment; the complexities interlacing proximity to others and exposure of the "self"; and the overwhelming social emptiness that accompanies it; all the while recognising, the creative, empowering and hopeful ways people live with, cope with and embody their anxious distress. It is to these experiences that this book now turns.

Note

1 Andrews (2019) has demonstrated how these humanistic tendencies may be reconceived through a posthuman lens.

References

Andrews, G.J. (2018) *Non-Representational Theory & Health: The Health in Life in Space-Time Revealing*. Routledge. https://doi.org/10.4324/9781315598468
Andrews, G.J. (2019) 'Health geographies II: The posthuman turn', *Progress in Human Geography*, 43(6), pp. 1109–1119. https://doi.org/10.1177/0309132518805812

Andrews, G.J. (2021) 'Bios and arrows: On time in health geographies', *Geography Compass*, 15(4), p. e12559. https://doi.org/10.1111/gec3.12559

Atkinson, S. (2013) 'Beyond components of wellbeing: The effects of relational and situated assemblage', *Topoi*, 32(2), pp. 137–144. https://doi.org/10.1007/s11245-013-9164-0

Bankey, R. (2004) 'The agoraphobic condition', *Cultural Geographies*, 11(3), pp. 347–355. https://doi.org/10.1191/1474474004eu311ra

Benton, A., Sangaramoorthy, T., and Kalofonos, I. (2017) 'Temporality and positive living in the age of HIV/AIDS--A multi-sited ethnography', *Current Anthropology*, 58(4), pp. 454–476. https://doi.org/10.1086/692825

Blackman, L. and Venn, C. (2010) 'Affect', *Body & Society*, 16(1), pp. 7–28. https://doi.org/10.1177/1357034X09354769

Bodden, S. et al. (2022) *Winter worries: Understanding experiences of seasonal affective disorder in the UK through the 2022 'Big SAD Survey'*. Interim project report.

Boyd, C.P. (2017) *Non-Representational Geographies of Therapeutic Art Making*. Springer International Publishing. https://doi.org/10.1007/978-3-319-46286-8

Boyle, L. (2019) 'The (un)habitual geographies of social anxiety disorder', *Social Science & Medicine*, 231, pp. 31–37. https://doi.org/10.1016/j.socscimed.2018.03.002

Brijnath, B. and Antoniades, J. (2016) '"I'm running my depression:" Self-management of depression in neoliberal Australia', *Social Science & Medicine*, 152, pp. 1–8. https://doi.org/10.1016/j.socscimed.2016.01.022

Burke, E. (2006) 'Feminine visions: Anorexia and contagion in pop discourse', *Feminist Media Studies*, 6(3), pp. 315–330. https://doi.org/10.1080/14680770600802066

Campbell, R. and Longhurst, R. (2013) 'Obsessive–compulsive disorder (OCD): Gendered metaphors, blogs and online forums', *New Zealand Geographer*, 69(2), pp. 83–93. https://doi.org/10.1111/nzg.12011

Charmaz, K. (1983) 'Loss of self: A fundamental form of suffering in the chronically ill', *Sociology of Health & Illness*, 5(2), pp. 168–195. https://doi.org/10.1111/1467-9566.ep10491512

Chouinard, V. (2012) 'Mapping bipolar worlds: Lived geographies of "madness" in autobiographical accounts', *Health & Place*, 18(2), pp. 144–151. https://doi.org/10.1016/j.healthplace.2011.08.009

Coaten, M. (2022) 'Voice-hearing and lived space', in Woods, A., Alderson-Day, B. and Fernyhough, C. (eds.) Chapter 19. *Voices in Psychosis: Interdisciplinary perspectives*. Oxford University Press: Oxford.

Conradson, D. (2003) 'Geographies of care: Spaces, practices, experiences', *Social & Cultural Geography*, 4(4), pp. 451–454. https://doi.org/10.1080/1464936032000137894

Cromby, J. (2014) 'Embodiment', in T. Teo (ed.) *Encyclopedia of Critical Psychology*. New York, NY: Springer, pp. 550–555. https://doi.org/10.1007/978-1-4614-5583-7_89

Davidson, J. (2000) '"… the world was getting smaller": Women, agoraphobia and bodily boundaries', *Area*, 32(1), pp. 31–40.

Davidson, J. (2001) 'Fear and trembling in the mall: Women, agoraphobia, and body boundaries, in Dyck, I., Davis Lewis, N., and McLafferty, S. (eds.) *Geographies of Women's Health*. 1st Edition, Routledge: London, pp. 213–230.

Davidson, J. (2005) 'Contesting stigma and contested emotions: Personal experience and public perception of specific phobias', *Social Science & Medicine*, 61(10), pp. 2155–2164. https://doi.org/10.1016/j.socscimed.2005.04.030

De Timary, P., Heenen-Wolff, S., and Philippot, P. (2011) 'The question of "representation" in the psychoanalytical and cognitive-behavioral approaches. Some theoretical aspects and therapy considerations', *Frontiers in Psychology*, 2, pp. 1–8. https://doi.org/10.3389/fpsyg.2011.00071

Del Casino Jr, V.J. (2007) 'Health/sexuality/geography' in Browne, K., Lim, J., and Brown, G. (eds.) *Geographies of Sexualities* Chapter 3. Routledge: London.

Driedger, S.M., Crooks, V.A. and Bennett, D. (2004) 'Engaging in the disablement process over space and time: Narratives of persons with multiple sclerosis in Ottawa, Canada', *The Canadian Geographer / Le Géographe canadien*, 48(2), pp. 119–136. https://doi.org/10.1111/j.0008-3658.2004.00051.x

Duff, C. (2016) 'Atmospheres of recovery: Assemblages of health', *Environment and Planning A: Economy and Space*, 48(1), pp. 58–74. https://doi.org/10.1177/0308518X15603222

Espeso, C.S.-R. (2022) 'From safe places to therapeutic landscapes: The role of the home in panic disorder recovery', *Wellbeing, Space and Society*, 3, p. 100108. https://doi.org/10.1016/j.wss.2022.100108

Evans, J. (2018) 'De-centering geographies of health: The challenge of post-structuralism', in V.A. Crooks, G.J. Andrews, and J. Pearce (eds) *Routledge Handbook of Health Geography*. London: Routledge.

Evans, J. and Wilton, R. (2019) 'Well enough to work? Social enterprise employment and the geographies of mental health recovery', *Annals of the American Association of Geographers*, 109(1), pp. 87–103. https://doi.org/10.1080/24694452.2018.1473753

Fang, C. et al. (2023) '"I am just a shadow of who I used to be"—Exploring existential loss of identity among people living with chronic conditions of Long COVID', *Sociology of Health & Illness*. https://doi.org/10.1111/1467-9566.13690

Gesler, W.M. (1992) 'Therapeutic landscapes: Medical issues in light of the new cultural geography', *Social Science & Medicine*, 34(7), pp. 735–746. https://doi.org/10.1016/0277-9536(92)90360-3

Gibson, K., Moffatt, S., and Pollard, T.M. (2022) '"He called me out of the blue": An ethnographic exploration of contrasting temporalities in a social prescribing intervention', *Sociology of Health & Illness*, 44(7), pp. 1149–1166. https://doi.org/10.1111/1467-9566.13482

Hall, E. (2000) '"Blood, brain and bones": Taking the body seriously in the geography of health and impairment', *Area*, 32(1), pp. 21–29.

Holmes, J. (2008) 'Space and the secure base in agoraphobia: A qualitative survey', *Area*, 40(3), pp. 375–382. https://doi.org/10.1111/j.1475-4762.2008.00820.x

Ireland, A.V. et al. (2019) 'Walking groups for women with breast cancer: Mobilising therapeutic assemblages of walk, talk and place', *Social Science & Medicine*, 231, pp. 38–46. https://doi.org/10.1016/j.socscimed.2018.03.016

Johnstone, L. and Boyle, M. (2020) *The power threat meaning framework: Towards the identification of patterns in emotional distress, unusual experiences and troubled or troubling behaviour, as an alternative to functional psychiatric diagnosis.*

Jowsey, T. (2016) 'Time and chronic illness: A narrative review', *Quality of Life Research*, 25(5), pp. 1093–1102. https://doi.org/10.1007/s11136-015-1169-2

Jowsey, T. et al. (2016) 'Time to manage: Patient strategies for coping with an absence of care coordination and continuity', *Sociology of Health & Illness*, 38(6), pp. 854–873. https://doi.org/10.1111/1467-9566.12404

Kearns, R.A. (1993) 'Place and health: Towards a reformed medical geography*', *The Professional Geographer*, 45(2), pp. 139–147. https://doi.org/10.1111/j.0033-0124.1993.00139.x

Kearns, R.A. (1995) 'Medical geography: Making space for difference', *Progress in Human Geography*, 19(2), pp. 251–259. https://doi.org/10.1177/030913259501900206

Kearns, R.A. and Gesler, W.M. (1998) *Putting Health into Place: Landscape, Identity, and Well-being*. Syracuse, NY: Syracuse University Press.

Kelly, M. (2010) 'Who cares............for the carers?', *Journal of Renal Care*, 36(1), pp. 16–20. https://doi.org/10.1111/j.1755-6686.2010.00139.x

Kidd, A.N. and MacArthur, K.S. (2019) 'Happy affect: Harnessing chance and uncertainly in design practice', *The Design Journal*, 22(sup1), pp. 1747–1760. https://doi.org/10.1080/14606925.2019.1594937

Laketa, S. and Côte, M. (2023) 'Discomforts in the academy: From "academic burnout" to collective mobilisation', *Gender, Place & Culture*, 30(4), pp. 574–587. https://doi.org/10.1080/0966369X.2021.2014405

Laurier, E. and Philo, C. (2006) 'Possible geographies: A passing encounter in a café', *Area*, 38(4), pp. 353–363. https://doi.org/10.1111/j.1475-4762.2006.00712.x

Laws, J. (2009) 'Reworking therapeutic landscapes: The spatiality of an "alternative" self-help group', *Social Science & Medicine*, 69(12), pp. 1827–1833. https://doi.org/10.1016/j.socscimed.2009.09.034

Laws, J. (2013) '"Recovery work" and "magic" among long-term mental health service-users', *The Sociological Review*, 61(2), pp. 344–362. https://doi.org/10.1111/1467-954X.12020

Lea, J., Cadman, L. and Philo, C. (2015) 'Changing the habits of a lifetime? Mindfulness meditation and habitual geographies', *cultural geographies*, 22(1), pp. 49–65. https://doi.org/10.1177/1474474014536519

Leder, D. (1992) 'Introduction', in D. Leder (ed.) *The Body in Medical Thought and Practice*. Dordrecht: Springer Netherlands (Philosophy and Medicine), pp. 1–12. https://doi.org/10.1007/978-94-015-7924-7_1

Leys, R. (2011) 'The turn to affect: A critique', *Critical Inquiry*, 37(3), pp. 434–472. https://doi.org/10.1086/659353

Lucas, G. (2022) 'Moving matters: Living in the body after anorexia', in H. Lewis et al. (eds) *The Practical Handbook of Eating Difficulties: A Comprehensive Guide from Personal and Professional Perspectives*. Shoreham-by-Sea: Pavilion, pp. 331–338.

Lucherini, M. (2020) 'Spontaneity and serendipity: Space and time in the lives of people with diabetes', *Social Science & Medicine*, 245, p. 112723. https://doi.org/10.1016/j.socscimed.2019.112723

Marcum, J.A. (2005) 'Biomechanical and phenomenological models of the body, the meaning of illness and quality of care', *Medicine, Health Care and Philosophy*, 7(3), pp. 311–320. https://doi.org/10.1007/s11019-004-9033-0

Martin, E. (2021) *Mental ill-health and experiences of work in a 'working community' in Scotland*. Unpublished PhD Thesis. University of Glasgow, Scotland.

McGeachan, C. (2017) '"The Head Carver": Art extraordinary and the small spaces of asylum', *History of Psychiatry*, 28(1), pp. 58–71. https://doi.org/10.1177/0957154X16676693

McGrath, L., Reavey, P., and Brown, S.D. (2008) 'The scenes and spaces of anxiety: Embodied expressions of distress in public and private fora', *Emotion, Space and Society*, 1(1), pp. 56–64. https://doi.org/10.1016/j.emospa.2008.08.003

McQuoid, J., Jowsey, T., and Talaulikar, G. (2017) 'Contextualising renal patient routines: Everyday space-time contexts, health service access, and wellbeing', *Social Science & Medicine*, 183, pp. 142–150. https://doi.org/10.1016/j.socscimed.2017.04.043

McWade, B. (2015) 'Temporalities of mental health recovery', *Subjectivity*, 8(3), pp. 243–260. https://doi.org/10.1057/sub.2015.8

Mehta, A. and Bondi, L. (1999) 'Embodied discourse: On gender and fear of violence', *Gender, Place & Culture*, 6(1), pp. 67–84. https://doi.org/10.1080/09663699925150

Mezzalira, S. (2022) *'Trauma and Its Impacts on Temporal Experience: New Perspectives from Phenomenology and Psychoanalysis*. Routledge: New York.

Moss, P. (1997) 'Negotiating spaces in home environments: Older women living with arthritis', *Social Science & Medicine*, 45(1), pp. 23–33. https://doi.org/10.1016/S0277-9536(96)00305-X

Nieuwenhuis, M. and Knoll, E. (2021) 'Towards a geography of voice-hearing', *Emotion, Space and Society*, 40, p. 100812. https://doi.org/10.1016/j.emospa.2021.100812

Nilsen, G. and Elstad, I. (2009) 'Temporal experiences of persistent pain. Patients' narratives from meetings with health care providers', *International Journal of Qualitative Studies on Health and Well-being*, 4(1), pp. 51–61. https://doi.org/10.1080/17482620802416129

Orona, C.J. (1990) 'Temporality and identity loss due to Alzheimer's disease', *Social Science & Medicine*, 30(11), pp. 1247–1256. https://doi.org/10.1016/0277-9536(90)90265-T

Papoulias, C. and Callard, F. (2010) 'Biology's gift: Interrogating the turn to affect', *Body and Society*, 16(1), pp. 29–56. https://doi.org/10.1177/1357034X09355231

Parr, H. (1999) 'Delusional geographies: The experiential worlds of people during madness/illness', *Environment and Planning D: Society and Space*, 17(6), pp. 673–690. https://doi.org/10.1068/d170673

Parr, H. (2000) 'Interpreting the "hidden social geographies" of mental health: Ethnographies of inclusion and exclusion in semi-institutional places', *Health & Place*, 6(3), pp. 225–237. https://doi.org/10.1016/S1353-8292(00)00025-3

Parr, H. (2002a) 'Medical geography: Diagnosing the body in medical and health geography, 1999–2000', *Progress in Human Geography*, 26(2), pp. 240–251. https://doi.org/10.1191/0309132502ph367pr

Parr, H. (2002b) 'New body-geographies: The embodied spaces of health and medical information on the internet', *Environment and Planning D: Society and Space*, 20(1), pp. 73–95. https://doi.org/10.1068/d41j

Parr, H. (2006) 'Mental health, the arts and belongings', *Transactions of the Institute of British Geographers*, 31(2), pp. 150–166.

Parr, H. (2007) 'Mental health, nature work, and social inclusion', *Environment and Planning D: Society and Space*, 25(3), pp. 537–561. https://doi.org/10.1068/d67j

Parr, H. (2008) *Mental health and social space: towards inclusionary geographies?*, Wiley-Blackwell: London.

Parr, H., Philo, C., and Burns, N. (2003) '"That awful place was home":1 Reflections on the Contested Meanings of craig dunain asylum', *Scottish Geographical Journal*, 119(4), pp. 341–360. https://doi.org/10.1080/00369220318737183

Parr, H., Philo, C., and Burns, N. (2004) 'Social geographies of rural mental health: Experiencing inclusions and exclusions', *Transactions of the Institute of British Geographers*, 29(4), pp. 401–419. https://doi.org/10.1111/j.0020-2754.2004.00138.x

von Peter, S. (2010) 'The temporality of "Chronic" mental illness', *Culture, Medicine, and Psychiatry*, 34(1), pp. 13–28. https://doi.org/10.1007/s11013-009-9159-x

Philo, C. (2007) 'A vitally human medical geography? Introducing Georges Canguilhem to geographers', *New Zealand Geographer*, 63(2), pp. 82–96. https://doi.org/10.1111/j.1745-7939.2007.00095.x

Philo, C., Parr, H. and Burns, N. (2005) '"An oasis for us": "in-between" spaces of training for people with mental health problems in the Scottish Highlands', *Geoforum*, 36(6), pp. 778–791. https://doi.org/10.1016/j.geoforum.2005.01.002

Power, A. et al. (2019) '"Hopeful adaptation" in health geographies: Seeking health and wellbeing in times of adversity', *Social Science & Medicine*, 231, pp. 1–5. https://doi.org/10.1016/j.socscimed.2018.09.021

Rasmussen, D.M. and Elverdam, B. (2007) 'Cancer survivors' experience of time – time disruption and time appropriation', *Journal of Advanced Nursing*, 57(6), pp. 614–622. https://doi.org/10.1111/j.1365-2648.2006.04133.x

Rowles, G.D. (2000) 'Habituation and being in place', *The Occupational Therapy Journal of Research*, 20(1_suppl), pp. 52S–67S. https://doi.org/10.1177/15394492000200S105

Sakellariou, D., Nissen, N. and Warren, N. (2021) 'The lived temporalities of prognosis: Fixing and unfixing futures', *The Cambridge Journal of Anthropology*, 39(2), pp. 138–155. https://doi.org/10.3167/cja.2021.390210

Schlosser, A.V. (2018) '"They medicated me out": Social flesh and embodied citizenship in addiction treatment', *Contemporary Drug Problems*, 45(3), pp. 188–207. https://doi.org/10.1177/0091450918781590

Segrott, J. and Doel, M.A. (2004) 'Disturbing geography: Obsessive-compulsive disorder as spatial practice', *Social & Cultural Geography*, 5(4), pp. 597–614. https://doi.org/10.1080/1464936042000317721

Sharp, L.A. (2000) 'The Commodification of the Body and Its Parts', *Annual Review of Anthropology*, 29, pp. 287–328.

Simonsen, K. (2013) 'In quest of a new humanism: Embodiment, experience and phenomenology as critical geography*', *Progress in Human Geography*, 37(1), pp. 10–26. https://doi.org/10.1177/0309132512467573

Simopoulou, Z. and Chandler, A. (2020) 'Self-harm as an attempt at self-care', *European Journal for Qualitative Research in Psychotherapy*, 10, pp. 110–120.

Slatman, J. (2014) 'Multiple dimensions of embodiment in medical practices', *Medicine, Health Care, and Philosophy*, 17(4), 549–557. https://doi.org/10.1007/s11019-014-9544-2

Smith, N. (2012) 'Embodying brainstorms: The experiential geographies of living with epilepsy', *Social & Cultural Geography*, 13(4), pp. 339–359. https://doi.org/10.1080/14649365.2012.683806

Stevenson, O. (2016) 'Suicidal journeys: Attempted suicide as geographies of intended death', *Social & Cultural Geography*, 17(2), pp. 189–206. https://doi.org/10.1080/14649365.2015.1118152

Thien, D. (2005) 'After or beyond feeling? A consideration of affect and emotion in geography', *Area*, 37(4), pp. 450–454.

Tolia-Kelly, D.P. (2006) 'Affect: An ethnocentric encounter? exploring the "universalist" imperative of emotional/affectual geographies', *Area*, 38(2), pp. 213–217.

Toombs, S.K. (1990) 'The temporality of illness: Four levels of experience', *Theoretical Medicine*, 11(3), pp. 227–241. https://doi.org/10.1007/BF00489832

Tucker, I. (2010) 'Everyday spaces of mental distress: The spatial habituation of home', *Environment and Planning D: Society and Space*, 28(3), pp. 526–538. https://doi.org/10.1068/d14808

Tucker, I.M. and Lavis, A. (2019) 'Temporalities of mental distress: Digital immediacy and the meaning of "crisis" in online support', *Sociology of Health & Illness*, 41(S1), pp. 132–146. https://doi.org/10.1111/1467-9566.12943

Varlet, M. et al. (2014) 'Difficulty leading interpersonal coordination: Towards an embodied signature of social anxiety disorder', *Frontiers in Behavioral Neuroscience*, 8, p. 29. https://doi.org/10.3389/fnbeh.2014.00029

Vestman, C., Hasselroth, M. and Berglund, M. (2014) 'Freedom and confinement: Patients' experiences of life with home haemodialysis', *Nursing Research and Practice*, 2014, p. 252643. https://doi.org/10.1155/2014/252643

Wasson, S. (2021) 'Waiting, strange: Transplant recipient experience, medical time and queer/crip temporalities', *Medical Humanities*, 47(4), pp. 447–455. https://doi.org/10.1136/medhum-2021-012141

Wetherell, M. (2013) 'Affect and discourse – What's the problem? From affect as excess to affective/discursive practice', *Subjectivity*, 6(4), pp. 349–368. https://doi.org/10.1057/sub.2013.13

Williams, A. (2007) *Therapeutic Landscapes*. Ashgate.

Wilton, R.D. (1996) 'Diminished worlds? The geography of everyday life with HIV/AIDS', *Health & Place*, 2(2), pp. 69–83. https://doi.org/10.1016/1353-8292(95)00040-2

Wood, V.J. et al. (2015) '"Therapeutic landscapes" and the importance of nostalgia, solastalgia, salvage and abandonment for psychiatric hospital design', *Health & Place*, 33, pp. 83–89. https://doi.org/10.1016/j.healthplace.2015.02.010

Wyllie, M. (2005) 'Lived time and psychopathology', *Philosophy, Psychiatry, & Psychology*, 12(3), pp. 173–185. https://doi.org/10.1353/ppp.2006.0017

4 Temporal intensities

Ruminations and anticipations

Introduction

This chapter outlines the temporal "intensities" of social anxiety in order to examine the various ways that they are embodied and enacted as people orientate their social and spatial worlds. Intensities refer to the temporally varying forms and forces of social anxiety as it manifests bodily, asking how, materially and discursively, these manifestations texture participants' everyday lives. In order to understand the social and spatial implications of social anxiety explored in the substantive heart of this work, it is helpful to lay out the emotional and affective groundwork for understanding how social anxiety is variously embodied and indeed experienced *as* embodied. This chapter leans on psychoanalytically influenced work as a conceptual meeting point between temporal and affective worlds[1] (Pile, 2009a) (Chapter 3). I outline the temporalities and spatialities that shape the continuous interplay of "embodied affectivity" (Fuchs and Koch, 2014), an interplay firmly rooted in an emotional and sensorial continuum. Such *felt* dynamics emerge through states of anticipation, guilt, shame, humiliation, embarrassment and self-consciousness; and arise in/through the bodily signs and symptoms of anxiety, such as blushing, shaking, palpitations, sweating and stuttering. These states continuously punctuate experiential accounts and therefore, situating a discussion of such "intensities" at the beginning of the empirical narrative means that they will not need to be explicitly highlighted throughout the chapters that follow but should be held as ever-present factors throughout the remainder of this book.

These intensities have the effect of signalling, exacerbating and sustaining anxiety and are key components to understanding how social anxiety moulds and stifles social and spatial worlds. Furthermore, this chapter builds on Callard's (2003, p. 295) concerns about how to mediate the "palatable" version of psychoanalysis typically employed by human geographers, and present instead a psychoanalytically informed geography of social anxiety that centralises the individual prone "as much to inertia and repetition as to progressive transformation". The reality of social anxiety is all-consuming and one that is rarely "progressive" or "transformative", often rendering the individual liable to "repeat that [which] makes them suffer" (Van de Vijver, Bazan and Detandt, 2017, p. 1) through acts of

DOI: 10.4324/9781003206880-4

social avoidance, withdrawal and isolation. In this vein, I unearth the qualitative character of this experience, one that invariably, to use participants' words, "gets right under the skin", "weighs heavily", "paralyses", "cripples", "builds", "creeps", "seizes", "suffocates" and "invades"[2] their psychical and corporeal worlds. Crucially, this is not about locating a "root cause" of social anxiety in participants' personal histories, but rather about developing an understanding of how anxiety manifests, endlessly and relentlessly, in people's everyday social and spatial lives.

Psychoanalysis is fundamentally concerned with the coming into being of the subject, a process that is itself fraught with anxiety, and is conceptually relevant here for understanding how social anxiety ingrains itself into the life worlds of those experiencing it and maintains its "grip" on various aspects of their social and relational lives. Anticipation as an immanent property plays an important role in "identification" in terms of how our psyches are organised, how we orient ourselves in the world and how we distinguish between our inner and outer worlds. Yet, these processes do not start and end with identification.[3] As human beings, we are seemingly driven to find our place in the world by carrying out certain routines, practices and movements in order to find and then to maintain stability (Van de Vijver, 2000, p. 166; Davidson, 2003; Lucherini, 2016). Lacan stresses that the anticipatory processes of the subject are "constructed in two suspected motions" (Van de Vijver, 2000): one of time and one of space. A psychoanalytic approach to anticipatory processes prioritises the ever-evolving relationship between the self-body-world, cast as one that inexorably unfolds in relation to the subject's past experiences and (anticipated) futures. I attend to these dynamics beginning with what is termed "the aftermath" of an event, or "retroactivity", which will provide a clearer understanding of future-oriented anticipations in the context of social anxiety, before casting attention back on participant's repetitive ruminations. As such, this approach opposes the linear notion of subjective time and space, aiming to trace a conceptual path that tolerates and values the uncertainties and ambiguities that emerge in the ordinary complexities of social and spatial life.

Retroactivity

In order to understand the complexities of anticipatory processes, we start retroactively, in the *aftermath* of the event – a typically adverse event that may be subsequently experienced as traumatising. The reason for starting *afterwards* is perhaps not immediately obvious, particularly when anticipation lends itself *towards* an event. The notion of retroactivity serves an important and logical purpose concerning the "affective awakenings of the distant past" and their persistence in the present. Psychoanalytically, this *afterwardness*[4] concerns how an event "retroactively alters the subjective interpretation of the past" (Bistoen, Vanheule and Craps, 2014, p. 672). It is crucial for understanding not only the reality of the adversities that unfold throughout a person's life but how "the subject responded or reacted to this experience" and how that response "determined the effects of the so-called traumatic encounter." Verhaeghe (2012, p. 110) argues that "what is 'previous' comes into existence retroactively starting from the 'next'". This retroactive practice encompasses not only how past experiences are projected towards the future, thus influencing the "present" but also how "present" experiences influence the perception and interpretation of past events.[5] Psychoanalytic insights enable this experience of being "drawn back" to be conceptualised as a "return to", or repetition of, an earlier event. As such, these experiences, whether or not they actually happened in the manner in which they are consciously/unconsciously catalogued, are often problematically and devastatingly re-experienced in the present.

Lacan's psychoanalytic theory regards the unconscious as structured like a language (Lacan, 1988, p. 48). He argues that a word is only given sense and meaning by the word(s) that precede it, and a similar process can be attributed to events: *event 1* influences ("anticipates") the experience of *event 2*; while *event 2* retroactively *re*shapes the meaning and experience of *event 1*; *event 3* is subsequently influenced by the *re*shaping of *event 1* and the experience of *event 2*; then *event 3* retroactively works to *re*shape *event 1 and event 2*; and so on. Therefore, not only are past experiences, for example, childhood experiences, central to how one anticipates and interprets subsequent life events, but current experiences can influence the recall and interpretation of previous experiences and memories. There are many external intrusions – with different temporalities – significant to social anxiety that impose on the individual and have a lasting impact on the psyche. First, there are those that entail continuous and repeated exposure to interpersonal hostility and aggression (e.g. bullying or physical and/or emotional abuse); then, there are "micro-events", a series of separate events of a similar quality (e.g. isolated experiences of embarrassment or social exclusion); and finally, there are what may be considered "less severe stressors", ones not immediately recognisable as traumatic, but which can cause long-term mental and emotional distress (e.g. sudden changes in environment or ongoing experiences of stress) (Bisteon *et al.*, 2014). Such events, whether of instantaneous trauma or a regular feature in one's everyday life, serve as a form of "socio-symbolic violence" that operate as "brutal interruptions that destroy the symbolic texture of [a] subject's identity" (Žižek, 2011, p. 292).[6]

Psychoanalysis contends that event-encounters are internalised and inscribed and catalogued at a psychical level through processes of repression[7]; the "memories" of which are very much anchored in/to the body[8] (Pile, 2009b) and re-emerge in situations – in specific times and spaces – that are similar, in one form or another, to the "original" event. Crucially, memory does not function as a repository where experiences are stored, accessible and retrieved, but rather, like an archive, it is fragmented, pieced together and re-interpreted at a temporal and spatial disconnect. A complex process is at work in the recollection of memories, where recalled memories are comprised of precipitates and traces that are not necessarily representative of the original experience or event.[9] Memories may be distorted and distorting, but no less significant and signifying. Memory fragments are re-lived and re-embodied through practices of rumination and their forcible return into conscious thought, one where symptoms speak of a repression, absence and abundance (Hodder, 2017). Therefore, I attend to individual and private memories as social and spatial "remains" (Jones, 2011) and "reversions"[10] (Philo, 2006). Crucially, psychoanalysis is less concerned with any putative "real" sequence of an individual's past such as, establishing objectively verifiable sequences of events, rather, it is concerned with "the past insofar as it is historicised in the present – historicised in the present because it was lived in the past" (Lacan, 1991, p. 12). This implies an understanding that past events continue to be relevant and actively participate in the construction of meaning and identity in the present. Thus, the retroactive processes involved are symbolically related to being "stuck in the aftermath" of an event, one where past events (and their associated memories and bodily resonances) always return with an uncanny and uncertain familiarity.[11]

In the questionnaire responses, participants often refer to feelings such as being "stuck" (Jane, QR) or "trapped" (Kim, QR) by their anxiety,[12] while one of the most common expressions that participants use to describe what it is like to live with social anxiety is "a vicious cycle [or] circle". Such descriptions frame repetitions not as unproblematically formative practices that ensure continuity and instil belonging (Edensor, 2006), but as embodied events that continually burden, disturb, distress and isolate. Freud (1914) asserts that the most basic model of mental life entails, against all therapeutic efforts and interventions, the unconscious compulsion to repeat, since it is through repetition that we come to understand past events and experiences of trauma (Blum and Secor, 2011). Such circuitous loops are not only compulsive but also often counterproductive, representing "the perpetual recurrence of the same thing" (Freud, 1920, p. 22)[13] and marking a(n un)conscious return to a qualitatively similar set of experiences. For example, Jane, who grew up in an "authoritarian" household, describes how numerous events actively "condition" (in the present) her intense and vivid response to external "triggers", continuously serving to "send me back to my childhood":

> Imagine living with a military commander [her stepfather] who watches your every move, criticises everything and over-reacts to everything. Plus, the constant threats of violence and [a] disgusting sexual taint to everything. Although no physical violence or otherwise happened to me, the shouting, attacking furniture and having my bedroom ripped to shreds; the threat of everything melted my brain. [...] I find myself reacting overly fearfully to people [who] raise their voices because of the way my stepfather used to shout, especially with people who are authority figures – which is pretty much everyone because I feel lesser than everyone – I sort of sink into myself and withdraw.

Significant in Jane's discussion of her early memories are notions of being visible, of being watched, scrutinised and receiving a negative response from her stepfather, aspects that continue to have a pervasive impact on her daily life and form the very foundation of her experience with social anxiety. By internalising the authoritative, aggressive and threatening conditions that were a habitual feature in her early and formative years, Jane repeatedly re-experiences the feelings of uncertainty, anxiety and hostility in her current interpersonal and social relations. She also discusses how these traumatic memories are deeply tied to and embedded in places that command repetition[14]: "previous places where I've had bad times are a trigger too, for example if I walk by my secondary school, that can taint my social interactions for the rest of the day because I keep remembering negative stuff." The intrusive and uncontrollable repetition of "traumatic" experiences, maybe triggered by particular place-encounters, is often inescapable and prevents the individual from moving past them.

The surfacing of anxieties in particular interactions and situations that are symbolically reminiscent of the original event(s) demonstrates the (un)bound-edness of the psyche (Parr, 1999) and its often-problematic materialisation in the present. Kim describes three situations throughout her life that resurface when she encounters similar situations in the present:

K: I find myself remembering and kind of reliving all the times I messed up in important or significant situations and looked/felt like an idiot. Things that happened recently to things that happened 10 or 20 years ago

L: What interactions/situations do you remember?

K: I was bullied by co-workers and feel to some extent I let it happen/deserved it. It was easy for me to become the butt of their jokes/taunts. In school, messing up presentations, awkward exchanges with class-mates [and] being singled out and absolutely humiliated by a teacher for getting something wrong. [Then,] the time my mum tried to take me to dancing lessons and I freaked out. I was 5 or 6 at that time, but I remember all these details so vividly, I remember feeling so over-whelmed that it was painful and that's the same feeling I get time and time again like I'm stuck in my 5 or 15 or 20 year-old brain and body and I can't escape.

These memories resurface as fragments but their most salient points remain. Kim, now aged 25, tracks back from the most recent event, through her teen-age years to the overwhelmingly "painful" childhood memory where she was faced with the threat of performance. Her testimony, although brief, illumi-nates how various elements of her past (and present) experience are representa-tive of what went before, organised around themes of performance, humiliation, authority and confrontation, and situated in formative social environments. When I query Kim's (IR) reasoning for feeling that she deserved to be bullied or taunted, she replies saying, "Tbh,[15] my self-worth is so low that it was easier to take it than complain, plus, how was I going to bring that to my boss and then HR[16] and still have to face them every day? I couldn't go through that scrutiny." Eventually, she quit her job in an effort to escape the hostile work environment, but it is a situation to which she is effectively forced to return time and time again. Similar to Jane, Kim alludes to fears of authority figures. Throughout Kim and Jane's testimonies, and the testimonies of other participants, a relationship between social anxiety and the "situated" self emerges. The (past) sites and settings of traumatic and anxious events shed are constantly reiterated throughout Kim's and others' life course, profoundly affecting their sense of self and self-other-world relations.

Anticipations

Social anxiety is typically considered to be future-orientated, concerned with the *what if* of that which has not happened *yet*. Anticipation is fundamental to the shaping and sustaining of social anxieties, but this role is ambiguous and paradoxical. On the one hand, anticipation plays an important role as a structuring function in the coming-into-being of the subject (Van de Vijver, 1998): first, in terms of the "situatedness" of self in relation to others and the social world; and second, as a necessary function for taking "abstract" ideas and previous experiences and projecting them on to future beings and doings. On the other hand, the emotional and affective dimensions of anticipatory anxieties mark the "emergence of unpredictability" (Grosz, 2013, p. 225). Reliving the intensities of past and traumatic experiences not only seizes the individual but initiates the anxiety-drenched anticipations of a future that is continually encroaching on the present. The subject's forward projections and the impending nature of future threats inevitably meet, situating the subject in a space of subjective annihilation or existential dread.

Overwhelming and intolerable levels of anxiety cause significant anguish and emotional distress for the individual who is engulfed by memories of negative past experiences, and hence also by the threat of those experiences repeating:

> It's not just before, the anticipation. And it's not just during, the anxiety during the event. It's the after too. Social interactions from months ago I still haven't let go of. How I was perceived. Whether I wanted to be perceived that way (most the time no). It pulls me down because all social interactions make me feel bad about myself. Not Good Enough. Stupid. Selfish. Pathetic. Wrong. All of those negative judgements that I think of myself, and I perceive others are thinking of me, stick with me for a long time, if not forever.
>
> (Amelia, QR)

Amelia captures the overwhelming and distressing dynamics of anticipatory processes that are experienced before, during and after the social "event". Before an event, many participants describe experiencing a gradual accumulation of worry and uncertainty about potential and unknown futures. Crucially, while avoidant behaviours are common, many people endure social situations despite the intense levels of distress they experience. During such situations,

Amelia experiences a visceral feeling of vulnerability, causing intense aware-ness of the self and socio-spatial surroundings. After an event, many engages in a repetitive focus on issues relating to social performance and self-worth. The vision of the future and the experience of the present are often incoherent, destabilising and wrought with uncertainty. The anticipatory processes involved are always contingent upon the overlapping and intertwining of corporeal, relational, temporal and spatial dynamics.

Amelia's account of how her anxiety manifests exemplifies a sense of antici-pation that is both continuous and cumulative:

> It builds and builds over a matter of days or weeks [...] I just can't control my thoughts, or see clearly, everything is foggy and gets increasingly intense and my body doesn't contain anything. I sweat, and blush, shake, stutter and it's like my anxiety is just oozing out for everyone to see. It's awful. I'm so ashamed of not being able to control this. I'm waking up every day and worrying about what will happen, who I will have to talk to and where I will have to go. Will the door go? Will the phone ring? At the end of the day I go over in my head every last detail of what I did, what I said, how I said it, what my face looked like, did I make enough eye contact and how were people reacting to me? I'm constantly ques-tioning myself, doubting myself, criticising myself then it starts all over again.

The intimate entwinement of the time-space interactions and everyday mate-rialities[17] that constitute anticipatory processes are cruelly apparent and plainly embodied in Amelia's testimony. Her account describes a "cumulative effect" that "builds and builds" over extended periods of time, the repetitive questioning of "what if..." and the list of bodily symptoms all reinforcing a sense of gathering uncertainty. The affective and emotional manifestations here of anticipation signify the impending loss of control and are "sensorially overwhelming, emotionally uncomfortable, socially stigmatising and so, dis-abling" (Davidson and Parr, 2010, p.63). Similarly, terms like "constantly" and "starts all over again" all point to a symbolically structured and continuous cycle of anticipatory anxiety, one that cannot but initiate a "new" cycle of repetition.

Catastrophic thinking entails the imagining of worst-case scenarios, magni-fying immediate and eventual consequences of internal processes and external conditions regarded as threatening to the point of consuming the bounded self (Gellatly and Beck, 2016). Anderson states that it is through the act of imagin-ing that "futures are made present in affects, epistemic objects and materiali-ties" (2010, p. 779). On the one hand, individuals draw on external cues magnifying the perceived threat from others; and, on the other, they shift atten-tion to internal cues and warning signs (e.g. sensations, thoughts and emo-tions) that are interpreted as imminent signs of personal and social catastrophe. The perceived lack of control over the self and one's socio-spatial surroundings reinforces the belief that they cannot "do any of the normal social things re-quired to be a functioning human being" (Amelia, QR). John also notes simi-lar thought processes:

> Visually seeing a worst-case scenario in your head. So when my anxiety is at its worst I will actually imagine myself being around other people and having a full-blown panic attack and ending up in the hospital with [doctors] saying 'yes you're going crazy'. These things make my anxiety even worse and those thoughts just spiral out of control.
>
> (John, QR)

Participants frequently reference living with persistent feelings of "dread" or "losing control" which is commonly associated with losing physical control of bodily processes and, including "stomach churning, needing the toilet, sweat-ing [and] headaches", (Anya, QR), while others report "palpitations, leg tremor, facial twitching, sweating, blushing, sweaty palms, headaches, bodily/ muscle tension, jaw clenching, disturbed sleep (waking up early in the night and unable to get back to sleep) [and] mental/physical fatigue" (Simon, QR). Jane writes that because she "exists" in a constant state of anticipation:

> It is rare I feel truly relaxed or happy. I can't really enjoy things, they just don't attract me and I feel so little from them because I'm always so wor-ried [...] [and] socialising is so draining and difficult. Not being able to relax properly makes my tension worse as I can't unwind and the fear has me constantly winding tighter and tighter.

Ruminations

The most banal daily interactions can inflict cumulative psychical and emo-tional harm on the individual, with the minutiae of these interactions often the focus of self-conscious and self-critical practices of rumination conducted in the aftermath of an event.[18] Rumination manifests through habitually and "highly negative views of self and a painful and repetitive self-scrutiny [...] characterised by harsh internal dialogues about social performance or per-ceived failures" (Boyle, 2018, p. 2). This critical examination of the self in rela-tion to others compromises a person's self-other-world relations, frequently leading them to question their own social value and place in the world. In the aftermath, participants report feeling "worthless", "useless", "drained" and "dead inside",[19] wherein each repeated attempt to "be normal, live normally, have normal relationships with others and myself – just *live*" (Daniel, QR *emphasis added*) reinforces a sense of failure that produces a "less-than-human" (Philo, 2017) subject.

Daniel writes that he "spend[s] too much time analysing every interaction or situation" for social mistakes, faults or failings that, from his perspective, cause "other people to think negatively of [him]" (Daniel QR). In a follow-up interview, he describes the aftermath of a social event:

> Social things are stressful, I feel tense and nervous most of the time and I feel very self-conscious so they are pretty awful to deal with. When I am alone, I have all this time to sit with myself and run through everything I did or said, [to] worry about what other people think about me. I play it over and over and over again in my head. I really start to hate myself and how awkward and incapable I am of being normal in social situations. It spirals out of control and I can't stop thinking about it.

> L: What sort of things do you think about?
> D: I go over and over everything I said and did: Why I did it? How I did it? Why I did it that way? How I said something? (e.g. tone of voice, volume, projection, wording); How my body language or general demeanour makes me look anxious and weird and completely unapproachable – I feel people avoid me anyway because of this. I really beat myself up over being so unapproachable.
> L: When you have those conversations with yourself, how do you feel?
> D: Worthless. Beyond worthless. I've done nothing with my life and I feel so pitiful and empty. I've heard those thought patterns called 'analysis paralysis' and 'post-mortem' thinking, or something like that, but I feel like I'm already socially paralysed by them, I just exist; a lifeless existence.

Similar to the aforementioned retroactive events, practices of rumination have the capacity to "paralyse" the individual, cementing them in past interactions, sites and spaces. Daniel's "lifeless existence" can be compared to the notion of "social death", which Králová (2015) situates in direct opposition to "wellbeing" and notes that it is concerned with three interrelated socio-spatial conditions – loss of social identity, the loss of connection and social relations, and the disintegration of the body – which culminate in the individual's disconnection from social and spatial life. Amber (QR), meanwhile, describes her social anxiety as "crippling":

> It leaves me with a constant feeling of dread and unable to relax for any sustained period. My mind constantly recalls bad memories at the most random [times] which invokes hours/days more of self-criticism and feelings of wasted worthlessness. The majority of the time I feel like I just want to escape from everything and everyone and just exist alone.

Dean recalls that feeling like a "misfit" throughout his school years was shaped by others' perceptions of his character, which hindered his ability to maintain social connections and relationships:

I've never really fit in anywhere. I've always been a bit of a loner and a loser. I didn't fit in at school [and] any "friends"[20] I did have drifted or moved away. I often think about how painful those experiences were, all the times people gave me funny looks [when I was] trying to strike up a conversation with [them] – I was never really teased or anything, they just ignored me – [and] how dismissive teachers were of me. I feel society is equally dismissive now. They see me as this lonely weirdo.

Rumination, therefore, involves a conscious yet uncontrollable undoing of the (past) self in the present, as in how Natalie's ruminative practices have chipped away and hollowed out her sense of self:

I feel like the 'social' world drains the life out of me to be honest. It's so physically and mentally exhausting to try and stay tuned in to situations that are unbearable. I dwell on them endlessly, replaying the embarrassing interactions or awkward exchanges in my head. They are so intrusive and chip away at me. I feel like I've just become this shell of a person, you know?

This undoing of self often entails drawing comparisons to the self *before* it was gripped by social anxiety. Other participants reflect on their past selves with a feeling of sadness and loss for who "I used to be" (Karen, IR). *Becoming* socially anxious is often a slow and gradual process. Sarah comments that it "slowly infected" different areas of her social life and career, adding that, before she "had really got a hold on what was happening, it had completely wiped them out" (Sarah, IR). The practices of rumination raise questions about what constitutes continuity and coherence in/with the self, and signals the huge difficulties in trying to reconcile a new and "anxious" sense of self with a previously "more sociable" and specifically "unanxious" self. Loss of self and difficulties with identity were strongly related to perceptions of normality and living with "ill/well" selves.

Jess's testimony is difficult to situate under a specific heading of "retroactive", "rumination" or "anticipation" as she tracks back and forth through various times and spaces in an effort to "locate" her anxieties. I make no attempt here to restructure Jess's testimony into a more coherent narrative following a logical progression of "past-present-future". Rather, I want to emphasise the "bits and pieces, snapshots, grabs and glimpses of respondent lived experiences" (Vickers, 2012) through which various memories, times and spaces unfold in this singular act of reflection:

I can never quite put my finger on what it is that causes me to experience such crippling anxiety. I wasn't always like this. Is it that I might be laughed at? Is it that I might come across the wrong way? Is it that I'll show signs of anxiety or nervousness? All I know is that a whole host of innocuous situations, from going to the shops to making a telephone call to ordering a coffee, cause me to zero in on myself and analyse every aspect of the situation and myself in that situation, replaying how I think I appear to [others] in that moment. Weird, no doubt! [...] I actually just had to phone the doctor (tell me if this is useless info btw[21]) and it took me all morning and afternoon but I knew I had to do it before this [interview]. I could kick myself for the STATE I get myself into over making a fucking phone call ... [I'm thinking the receptionist at the doctors] will think: 'Oh, her again', 'what now?' and I got all flustered trying to make an appointment. Anyway. Sorry, I don't know how I got here to this point in my life.

(Jess, IR)

In the first instance, Jess is unable to place what came before her anxiety, but proceeds to project herself forward, anticipating the consequences of an imagined future, although one not outwith the realms of her experience. She connects her distressing anticipations with several everyday situations (e.g. shops, telephone and coffee), assuming that there will be an immediate and glaring "fault" or "failing", on which she "zero[s] in", selecting herself as target. Followed by a short account of making a telephone call several hours before our interview took place, she checks whether her experiential accounts are "useless" before she reflects on the morning's anticipations before reflexively "kicking herself" for being so overwhelmed by the seemingly simple task of making a doctor's appointment. She then ruminates over the receptionist's perceptions of her before cycling back round to her initial query: How did I get here? Or, from where did I get here? and why does what happened previously continuously disrupt what happens in the here and now?

Concluding remarks

This chapter lays the emotional and affective groundwork of anxious experiences that will be discussed at length in the following chapters. I explored the emotional and affective "intensities" of social anxiety in order to examine the various ways that they are embodied and enacted as people orientate their social and spatial worlds. I have sought to engage an understanding of how social anxiety is continuously structured and situated through the entwining temporalities and potentialities of anticipatory processes. Through these intensities, experienced as repetitions, ruminations, and anticipations, I consider the force and form of social anxiety and how materially and discursively these manifestations texture participants' everyday (and longer-term) lives and geographies. Despite the cyclical and pervasive repetition of anxious experiences, they are never seamlessly habituated, and rather they continue – as themselves habitually revisited, reappraised and consequential for routine decision-making – to rupture the fabric of everyday life and spaces. It is obvious that the affective and emotional dimensions of social anxiety cannot be readily separated from the sites and settings in which they are encountered or from the past memories, experiences and traumas that they are entangled with. The present continues to "present" the individual with repeating scenarios of a humiliated and shamed self, one that is always faltering and failing at the point of human connection or simply being human. The remnants of previous interpersonal and social encounters and events, forever relived, draw our attention to the inescapable situatedness of social life in a way that highlights what it means to be "unbearably human" (Philo, 2017, p. 260). The minutiae of daily life provide infinite fodder for critical, self-reflexive ruminations, for people with social anxiety. The intensities of experience depicted here point to processes and experiences that exhaust and confine, rather than enliven and liberate the individual, demonstrating how social anxiety so debilitatingly distresses and disrupts self-other-world relations.

Notes

1 While I draw on affective/non-representational geographies, many geographers in this domain would argue that the methodological approach implemented in this project has already rendered affect lost. This is where I feel a purely non-representational approach falls short, as to attempt to understand the nuances of social anxiety removed from the "speaking subject" (Wetherell, 2013) would restrict our understanding of how people *feel* and *embody* social anxiety, whether this be through the aforementioned intensities that cause feelings of precarity and insecurity to ensue or through internalising "pathologies" or societal norms and stigma.

2 These descriptions, and ones like them, that capture the embodied weight and presence of anxiety emerge continuously throughout participants' questionnaire and interview responses.

3 While many psychoanalysts look to childhood experiences to locate and unearth unconscious traumatic events, we continue to change and develop throughout our lives, it is imperative to look beyond exclusive childhood experiences and for "patients" to identify the ongoing sources of their anxieties.

4 From the Freudian concept of *"Nachträglichkeit"* (Lacan's *"apres coup"*) is central to his theories on trauma.

5 By "event", I mean a happening, memory and/or trauma significant to the individual.

6 A question posed to psychoanalysis is why the psychical consequences of, for example, two people with similar "traumatic" experiences may play out in completely different ways. Arguably, this rests on a host of internal and external factors and, ultimately, it is how these events are processed in relation to these factors that accounts for whether traumatic experiences re-emerge in the individual (or not).

7 Repression is one of the most fundamental principles of psychoanalysis and "denotes the process by which certain thoughts or memories are expelled from consciousness and confined to the unconscious" (Evans, 2006, p. 168).

8 Freud uses the term *"aufheben"*, which translates loosely "to suppress". Zizek uses the term "sublate" meaning "to assimilate (a smaller entity) into a larger one" (Oxford English Dictionary, n.d.). The latter attends to a "layering" of traumatic events that build, shift and manifest in other ways, where the events each have a qualitatively similar affect.

9 Laplanche (1999, p. 91) considers "the unconscious element or trace *not as a stored memory or representation, but as a sort of waste-product of certain processes of memorisation"*.

10 A local or temporary return to a previous state or practice: cf. "regression", a long-term return to an earlier, usually childhood, state (Bever, 2017).

11 Freud (1919, p. 245) states that "the uncanny is something which is *secretly familiar*, which has underdone repression and then returned from it".

12 Interestingly, while many feel "stuck" and "trapped" by their social anxieties, one of the biggest sources of anxiety about navigating everyday environments is a fear of *not* being able to escape. This is evident when participants discuss being in various social or public spaces and, in particular, on public transport (Chapter 7) and this lack of progressive movement is arguably also in play here.

13 This material is the ultimate focus of psychoanalytic therapy.

14 "The very mode of this determining is overdetermined by the present synchronous symbolic network. If the trace of an old encounter all of a sudden begins to exert an impact, it is because the present symbolic universe of the subject is structured in a way that is susceptible to it" (Žižek, 1991, p.202).

15 Short-hand for "to be honest".

16 Human Resources.

17 In the remainder of this book (Chapters 5, 6, 7 and 8), I highlight how the materialities of various mundane objects and spaces (e.g. telephones, doorbells, waiting rooms and corridors) are anticipatory.

18 In cognitive-behavioural approaches, this is referred to as "post-mortem thinking".

19 Numerous respondents.

20 Dean says he writes "friends", as any friends he did have were a product of the environment, that is "kids forced together at school or my mum's friend's kids."

21 Shorthand for "by the way". Side-notes like this one appeared regularly in the questionnaire responses and in conversations with participants, who were unconvinced of the "value" or "usefulness" of their stories. This, in itself, portrays a certain situational anxiety and highlights an arguably heightened self-conscious awareness in questionnaire and interview settings.

References

Anderson, B. (2010) 'Preemption, precaution, preparedness: Anticipatory action and future geographies', *Progress in Human Geography*, 34(6), pp. 777–798. https://doi.org/10.1177/0309132510362600

Bever, T.G. (2017) *Regressions in Mental Development: Basic Phenomena and Theories*. London: Routledge.

Bistoen, G., Vanheule, S., and Craps, S. (2014) '*Nachträglichkeit*: A Freudian perspective on delayed traumatic reactions', *Theory & Psychology*, 24(5), pp. 668–687. https://doi.org/10.1177/0959354314530812

Blum, V. and Secor, A. (2011) 'Psychotopologies: Closing the circuit between psychic and material space', *Environment and Planning D: Society and Space*, 29(6), pp. 1030–1047.

Boyle, L.E. (2018) 'The (un)habitual geographies of Social Anxiety Disorder', *Social Science & Medicine* [Preprint]. https://doi.org/10.1016/j.socscimed.2018.03.002

Callard, F. (2003) 'The taming of psychoanalysis in geography', *Social & Cultural Geography*, 4(3), pp. 295–312.

Davidson, J. (2003) *Phobic Geographies: The Phenomenology and Spatiality of Identity*. London: Routledge. https://doi.org/10.4324/9781315246864

Davidson, J. and Parr, H. (2010) 'Enabling cultures of dis/order online', in V. Chouinard, E. Hall, and R. Wilton (eds) *Towards Enabling Geographies: 'Disabled' Bodies and Minds in Society and Space*. Surrey: Ashgate Publishing, pp. 63–84.

Edensor, T. (2006) 'Reconsidering National Temporalities: Institutional Times, Everyday Routines, Serial Spaces and Synchronicities', *European Journal of Social Theory*, 9(4), pp. 525–545. https://doi.org/10.1177/1368431006071996

Evans, D. (2006) *An Introductory Dictionary of Lacanian Psychoanalysis*. London: Taylor & Francis.

Freud, S. (1914) 'Remembering, repeating and working-through: Further Recommendations on the Technique of Psychoanalysis II', in J. Riviere (tran.) *Collected Papers Vol. 2*, pp. 336–376. London: Hogarth Press.

Freud, S. (1919) 'The "Uncanny"', in Strachey, J. (ed) *The Standard Edition of the Complete Psychological Works of Sigmund Freud, Volume XVII [1917-1919]: An Infantile Neurosis and Other Works*, pp. 217–256. London: Hogarth Press.

Freud, S. (1920) *Beyond the Pleasure Principle*. https://www.sigmundfreud.net/beyond-the-pleasure-principle-pdf-ebook.jsp (Accessed: 4 April 2018).

Fuchs, T. and Koch, S.C. (2014) 'Embodied affectivity: On moving and being moved', *Frontiers in Psychology*, 5. https://doi.org/10.3389/fpsyg.2014.00508

Gellatly, R. and Beck, A.T. (2016) 'Catastrophic thinking: A transdiagnostic process across psychiatric disorders', *Cognitive Therapy and Research*, 40(4), pp. 441–452. https://doi.org/10.1007/s10608-016-9763-3

Grosz, E. (2013) 'Habit today: Ravaisson, Bergson, Deleuze and us', *Body & Society*, 19(2–3), pp. 217–239. https://doi.org/10.1177/1357034X12472544

Hodder, J. (2017) 'On absence and abundance: Biography as method in archival research', *Area (Oxford, England)*, 49(4), pp. 452–459. https://doi.org/10.1111/area.12329

Jones, O. (2011) 'Geography, memory and non-representational geographies', *Geography Compass*, 5(12), pp. 875–885. https://doi.org/10.1111/j.1749-8198.2011.00459.x

Králová, J. (2015) 'What is social death?', *Contemporary Social Science*, 10(3), pp. 235–248. https://doi.org/10.1080/21582041.2015.1114407

Lacan, J. (1988) *The Seminar of Jacques Lacan: Book 20 [XX]*. Edited by J.-A. Miller. New York: Norton.

Lacan, J. (1991) *The Seminar of Jacques Lacan: Book 1, Freud's Papers on Technique, 1953-1954*. Edited by J.-A. Miller. Translated by J. Forrester. New York: W. W. Norton & Company.

Laplanche, J. (1999) *Essays on Otherness*. New York: Psychology Press.

Lucherini, M. (2016) 'Performing diabetes: Surveillance and self-management', *Surveillance & Society*, 14(2), pp. 259–276. https://doi.org/10.24908/ss.v14i2.5996

Oxford English Dictionary (n.d.) *English Dictionary, Thesaurus, & grammar help | Oxford Dictionaries, Oxford Dictionaries | English*. https://en.oxforddictionaries.com/ (Accessed: 25 February 2019).

Parr, H. (1999) 'Delusional geographies: The experiential worlds of people during madness/illness', *Environment and Planning D: Society and Space*, 17(6), pp. 673–690.

Philo, C. (2006) 'Madness, memory, time, and space: The eminent psychological physician and the unnamed artist – Patient', *Environment and Planning D: Society and Space*, 24(6), pp. 891–917. https://doi.org/10.1068/d3305

Philo, C. (2017) 'Less-than-human geographies', *Political Geography*, 60, pp. 256–258. https://doi.org/10.1016/j.polgeo.2016.11.014

Pile, S. (2009a) 'Emotions and affect in recent human geography', *Transactions of the Institute of British Geographers*, 35(1), pp. 3–20. https://doi.org/10.1111/j.1475-5661.2009.00368.x

Pile, S. (2009b) 'Topographies of the body-and-mind: Skin Ego, Body Ego, and the film Memento', *Subjectivity*, 27(1), pp. 134–154.

Van de Vijver, G. (1998) 'Anticipatory systems a short philosophical note', *AIP*, pp. 31–37. https://doi.org/10.1063/1.56308

Van de Vijver, G. (2000) 'The Role of Anticipation in the Constitution of the Subject', in D.M. Dubois (ed.) *Computing Anticipatory Systems: CASYS'99 - Third International Conference*, pp. 161–167.

Van de Vijver, G., Bazan, A., and Detandt, S. (2017) 'The mark, the thing, and the object: On what commands repetition in Freud and Lacan', *Frontiers in Psychology*, 8. https://doi.org/10.3389/fpsyg.2017.02244

Verhaeghe, P. (2012) 'Lacan's answer to the classical mind/body deadlock: Retracing Freud's beyond', in S. Barnard and B. Fink (eds) *Reading Seminar XX: Lacan's Major Work on Love, Knowledge, and Feminine Sexuality*. New York: SUNY Press, pp. 109–140.

Vickers, M. (2012) 'Antenarratives to inform health care research: Exploring workplace illness disclosure for people with multiple sclerosis (MS)', *Journal of Health and Human Services Administration*, 35(2), p. 170.

Wetherell, M. (2013) 'Affect and discourse – What's the problem? From affect as excess to affective/discursive practice', *Subjectivity*, 6(4), pp. 349–368. https://doi.org/10.1057/sub.2013.13

Žižek, S. (2011) *Living in the End Times*. Verso.

5 Making sense of anxious experiences

Self-diagnosis, diagnosis and help-seeking

Introduction

Diagnosis is both a process and a category. As a medical process, it is "the thing that the physician does: the conclusion reached [and] the act of coming to that conclusion"; as a category, it concerns where that conclusion is situated within existing medical frameworks and in relation to specific causes, descriptions, sites and symptoms (Blaxter, 1978, p. 9). The function of diagnosis is also practical, administrative and symbolic: establishing, and enabling access to, specific courses of treatment and clearing a path towards "recovery"; enabling access to "service and status" (Jutel, 2009, p. 278), including sick leave and accommodations[1]; and for explaining, legitimising, providing relief, assigning meaning to, and giving permission to be, ill (Jutel 2009). Arguably, much has changed in the landscape of health and care since Blaxter's sociological intervention on diagnostic practice, and while it still holds true that medical diagnosis "forms the foundation of medical authority", it is also "contested, socially created, framed and/or enacted" (Jutel and Nettleton, 2011, p. 793).

Critical to this shift was an increasing awareness of the need to take "subjective interpretations of health [and illness] into account" (Prior, 2003, p. 42) and the increasing availability and accessibility of health and medical information online, which has not only impacted the doctor-patient relationship but dramatically enabled patient empowerment and engagement (Nettleton and Burrows, 2003). Equally, online communities, web forums and applications have become vital sources of immediate information, connection and support for people experiencing mental and emotional distress (Parr, 2002; Davidson and Parr, 2010; Campbell and Longhurst, 2013; Tucker and Lavis, 2019). This interaction between increased recognition of experience, increased accessibility and the ability to exchange information in supportive communities has established the role of the "expert patient" (Fox et al., 2005b), enabling people to participate meaningfully in their own health and care, accommodate different perspectives on health, promote self-management, resourcefulness and confidence, and advocate for themselves and others.

With this in mind, this chapter contends with how people experience, negotiate and participate in diagnosis, and how diagnosis and the practices of

DOI: 10.4324/9781003206880-5

help-seeking associated with it are "temporally and spatially complex" (Callard, 2014, p. 528). Caught up in these considerations is a concern with how conceptualisations of social anxiety – and mental and emotional distress more broadly – shape how people understand, negotiate and navigate such spaces and practices. Social anxiety continues to be conceptualised across a spectrum of social and medical perspectives, from normal human expressions of shyness, introversion and embarrassment to a serious mental disorder (Chapter 2); perspectives link to differing notions of personhood, identities and forms of self-governing. There is, of course, immense social power in diagnosis (Rosenberg, 2002). Embedded within it is a system of "social and cultural beliefs and meanings about the self and others, identity, normalcy and deviance, health and infirmity" (Ebeling, 2011, p. 831). Building from some of the issues raised in Chapter 2, concerned with the expanding scope of psychiatric diagnosis as a tool used to govern social and emotional lives, this chapter explores how diagnosis (by the self or other authorities) renders ongoing anxious distress intelligible and actionable. Relevant to this discussion is the narrowing of how we describe, diagnose and respond to distress, and how that narrowing ultimately filters back through people's experiences and conceptualisations of themselves and their anxiety, what Rose (2006, p. 480) describes as the "problem/solution complex", which:

> [...] simultaneously judges mood against certain desired standards, frames discontents in a certain way, renders them as a problem in need of attention, establishes a classification framework to name and delineate them, scripts a pattern of affects, cognitions, desires and judgements, writes a narrative for its origins and destiny, attributes it meaning, identifies some authorities who can speak and act wisely in relation to it and prescribes some responses to it.

These narratives provide people with the language to define their medical and emotional needs and potentially identify appropriate remedies. Even for those who find utility in or even subscribe to biomedical models, the "meaning" of their symptoms is "reduced to the properties that correspond to one category or box [and so] there is little space for personal meanings and personal narratives" (Stanghellini, 2004, p. 184) to be explored or taken into account. Thus, this chapter aims also to provide those accounts with context, to understand the meaning and significance of diagnosis-seeking, while also reflecting on the limitations of this process. Broadly, it addresses how understandings and experiences of social anxiety are inevitably caught up in medical, psychological and social discourses, and the various ways they are adopted, reinforced and/or resisted.

In order to proceed, this chapter maps the typically anxious journey of diagnosis and wider help-seeking. This provides a detailed picture of how diagnosis and the different interactions and spaces involved are encountered. First, examining the practice of self-diagnosis addresses how and why people seek out diagnosis and the meanings ascribed to their embodied experiences. This section also identifies the barriers that people face to formal diagnosis. It then briefly examines how the physical environment of various "healing" spaces shapes the experience of help-seeking. Overall, this gives a sense of how people with social anxiety obtain and apprehend their diagnosis within, alongside or outwith traditional mental healthcare pathways.

There are several reasons to focus on diagnosis, including self-diagnosis, and help-seeking practices of people with social anxiety. First, it is in stark recognition that 50% of socially anxious people will never seek help and support from healthcare professionals. The 50% who do so generally live with ongoing symptoms of distress for 15–20 years before taking this route (NICE, 2013, pp. 5–6). Moreover, not only are there potentially decades of lost time for those who fly "under the radar" and do not receive adequate or timely support; there are others marooned by their anxiety to such an extent that there is never any recourse to formal health and/or support systems for them. This lack of support precedes increased risk of social isolation, functional impairment, substance abuse, self-injury and suicidal thoughts and attempts (Olfson et al., 2000; Leigh et al., 2023). Therefore, it is imperative that healthcare profession-als and services possess an understanding of the extensive life experiences and histories (medical or otherwise) that people accumulate prior to engaging with health services, including histories of self-diagnosis, health literacy and exist-ing support systems, in order to provide adequate support alert to the multiple barriers people face in accessing adequate support and care.

Second, it is in recognition that many do not feel validated by their self-diagnosis or able to speak to their own experiences. This research invited those who had received a formal diagnosis and those who were self-diagnosed to participate, stating a clear focus on their lived experience regardless of "diag-nostic status". Despite this, several participants sought clarity on whether they were suitable participants for the research and for the follow-up online inter-views, because all they "had" was their own self-diagnosis:

> I've actually never been diagnosed with SA but I really identify with it and share very similar experiences to people on the forums, if this is use-ful to you, I'd like to participate.
>
> (Olivia, IR)

> I don't have a diagnosis yet. I'm in the process of trying to get one but it has been difficult. I'd like to take part in the interview if the lack of diag-nosis isn't an issue.
>
> (Brian, QR)

Kirsty[2] (QR) echoed similar concerns about whether her lack of "medical knowledge or technical terms" gave her authority to speak about her own experiences. Overall, this is clearly a population of people who have been largely ignored and feel let down by health professionals and mental health services. In spite of their social anxiety, they want to share their experiences and be recognised and understood, especially by those who they feel are often lacking in their ability to understand, empathise and provide appropriate support and resources for them.

Diagnosing the self

Self or lay diagnosis is a growing phenomenon, but one that is generally discouraged by medical institutions and patient organisations, except insofar as it may prompt subsequent engagement with health services. There are significant concerns about practices of self-diagnosis facilitated by the availability of health information online and the use of symptom checklists, self-assessments, screenings, quizzes and other "quasi-diagnostic" tools (Giles and Newbold, 2011). This concern has increased in recent years regarding diagnoses enabled, facilitated or perhaps proliferated, by artificial intelligence (AI) (Chen *et al.*, 2023); smartphone apps (Lupton and Jutel, 2015; Mackintosh *et al.*, 2020) and social media (Ross Arguedas, 2022). There are also concerns about misinformation that may lead to misdiagnosis, delayed treatment-seeking, or an alternative approach of self-management with recreational and/or over-the-counter drug use (Charlton, 2005) or result in increases in cyberchondria[3] (Starcevic and Berle, 2013). While recognised as collective sites of help-seeking, identity formation, community and resistance, online communities and social media have also been criticised for encouraging, romanticising and even glorifying certain harmful behaviours and illnesses, as in cases of "pro-ana" (pro-anorexia) and "pro-mia" (pro-bulimia) (Fox et al., 2005a), self-injury content (Boyd et al., 2011) and encouraging "pathological obsessions with healthy eating" in "orthorexia nervosa" (Ross Arguedas, 2022). Self-diagnosis can also be viewed in more positive terms as an "enactment of patient agency" (Ebeling, 2011, p. 829), one often associated with subverting medical logics (Ross Arguedas, 2022). In the context of social anxiety and as this section demonstrates, however, self-diagnosis can both appeal to and reject the dominant narratives that frame anxious distress as a "disorder", increasingly framed by biomedical and neurochemical logics (Rose 2003).

To give some context to the "diagnostic status" of participants in this research ($n = 130$): 48% ($n = 62$) were self-diagnosing with social anxiety; 50% ($n = 64$) report having received a formal diagnosis from a healthcare professional; 2% ($n = 2$) did not answer on this matter. Crucially, for those who had received a diagnosis from a healthcare professional, their diagnosis was, in almost all cases, preceded by self-diagnosis and enabled by lengthy information and help-seeking practices online.

The process of self-diagnosis typically begins online with a person connecting distressing thoughts, feelings and bodily symptoms to the diagnostic criteria of social anxiety, and/or to the shared experiences of others in online spaces, in a bid to try and make sense of the distress that they are experiencing:

> I typed some of my symptoms into Google and was led to a number of social anxiety sites, then onto the forum [SAUK].
> Self-diagnosing myself was a lightbulb moment for me.
> I had spent the better part of a decade thinking I was weird and abnormal for not wanting to or being able to socialise outside of school/work or hold onto friends. Reading the common features of SA, there were so many things which rang true for me. It was such a relief to be able to put a name to what I was feeling.
>
> (Lara, IR)

Identifying with social anxiety was a "lightbulb moment" that provided clarity and altered how Lara views herself, her experiences and her response to social situations. Being able to identify "that it's social anxiety" (Ben, QR) is noted as a critical step for many whether they went on to seek formal diagnosis or not. For some, self-diagnosis is a process of realisation; for others, it seems more intuitive and is attributed to an embodied self-awareness that they articulate as "just knowing". In an interview, Hannah says:

> When you live with something for long enough, you just know. I was incredibly anxious about very basic social interactions and it was ruining my life.
> I recognised that I was becoming more and more anxious about social life-related things and that got worse as time went on.
> Parties and stuff but then also interacting with family.
> I wasn't just nervous I was breaking down about very normal parts of daily life.
> "Social anxiety" just made sense and then I started researching it and realised it was a real thing and not just something I was making up.

Barriers to diagnosis and support

People's reasons for self-diagnosing vary but inevitably are caught up in the wider barriers faced in accessing more formal mental healthcare and support. At a fundamental level, seeking a diagnosis is a social encounter, one that entails telephone and face-to-face interactions with others, particularly with perceived authority figures (i.e. doctors and other healthcare staff), discussing personal and difficult situations and being in "clinical" spaces, all of which provoke and exacerbate anxiety (see below). Those who did not seek a diagnosis or who delayed treatment-seeking did so due to a number of interacting perceptual, practical, structural and occasionally geographical barriers. Overwhelmingly, a person's ability to seek further help was constrained by more practical concerns that lie at the heart of social anxiety, leaving the person at an impasse precisely because the help and support that they require necessitates interacting with others:

> I am simply too afraid to talk to my doctor. I can't even bear to pick up the phone to make an appointment let along *go* to the doctor's about it.
>
> (Natalie, QR)

> I know deep down I need to see a therapist and that I'd probably benefit from it but I literally don't know where to start. I don't even know what I would say without sounding ridiculous, "hi I'm scared to leave my house in case someone looks at me". I am scared bc[4] I don't want people paying attention to me or looking at me and that's basically what a therapy appointment is all about.
>
> (Rob, IR)

Similar experiences can be seen in those who self-diagnose autism spectrum disorder, in which social anxiety can be a significant factor and where the severity of anxiety impacts whether people will be able to make, attend and go through with an appointment to receive a formal diagnosis (Lewis, 2017). Perceptual barriers revolve around concerns about healthcare professionals "not believing me" (Simon, QR), "not taking me seriously [and] dismissing it" or not being "considered unwell enough" (Lara, QR) to warrant care and attention. Similarly, negative experiences with mental health services or health professionals including a lack of knowledge about social anxiety and feeling misunderstood can lead to feelings of distrust:

> *Beth:*   I self-diagnosed and haven't been diagnosed by a doctor and probably won't be.
>   I saw a doctor about my depression a number of years ago and his explanation was very "medical".
> *Louise:* What do you mean by 'medical'?
> *Beth:*   Like, no focus on my experience.
>   It was very much depression = a broken leg approach, so I guess I'm reluctant to [seek a formal diagnosis for social anxiety] because it's likely to be the same and I need an something that's a bit more focused on my past experiences. How it actually affects my life, sort of thing.

I asked Beth why she thought the broken leg analogy was problematic to which she replied:

> Well, it's just not accurate, is it? I get it in the sense that, y'no, it shouldn't be shameful and if I broke my leg I wouldn't *not* go to the hospital but

you can't bandage up the crippling anxiety I feel about day to day inter-actions and it won't heal on its own.

I just think the broken leg analogy paints a picture of knowing how to fix a broken leg, what recovery looks like, what therapies work, what medication will reduce the pain. There is a big difference between being unwell for years, decades for me and other folk, and temporarily injured, y'no?

Access to appropriate care and support is also hampered by limited under-standing of social anxiety, limited mental health resources, and lengthy wait times for, or a complete lack of access to, therapeutic services. Amy's experi-ence highlights a number of structural and geographical barriers because of the requirements of her doctor and her rural location:

I haven't been diagnosed officially. I'm up in [rural Scottish village] and my nearest doctor is in [several villages away] so I'd need to get the bus and I just can't do that. I have phoned them about it before but they need me to come up and that's something I can't do right now.

L: They didn't offer alternatives or talk over the phone?
A: He [the doctor] wanted to like see me in person cos it's "mental health" he says. He did offer a home visit but I live with my fam-ily, there's no privacy. [...]
    I just said I'll think about it and that was it.

Parr and Philo (2003) highlight the fraught nature and perceived risks of rural healthcare where social proximity to family and a lack of privacy shape how, or indeed whether, care practices occur. Amy also adds that the support offered would be an online, self-administered cognitive behavioural therapy course, and so the idea that she could not access remote treatment options without first physically travelling to see the doctor "seems nonsensical" to her. There is an argument then, that:

When it comes to emotional and psychological problems, [...] people 'soldier on', often not discussing such things with neighbours and even family, partly to avoid the gossip and partly to avoid the perceived stigma that contact with formal services can bring.

(Parr and Philo 2003, 476)

Seeking formal diagnosis

As might be expected, the pathways to help-seeking for social anxiety are lay-ered and complex (Mackian, 2002). Many participants note that obtaining a formal diagnosis was arduous, with others saying that it "accomplished very little" (Anna, QR). While many seek a diagnosis to validate and make sense of distressing experiences, others are less concerned about an "official diagnosis" and "just desperately need support [and] someone to talk to" (Ash, QR). In this sense, the doctor is seen as a gatekeeper not necessarily to diagnosis *per se*, but to specific treatments and allowances including medications, therapies and sick leave (Jutel, 2010). People often seek help as a last resort after numerous episodes of "crisis and then, sort of, rebound" (Ash, QR) or if their social anxiety starts having particularly adverse effects, for example, when behaviour becomes "destructive" and some may be at risk of "really harming myself" (Chloe, QR) (Edge and MacKian, 2010). The process is not straightforward and often causes further upset and distress. There was frequent mention of "being passed from pillar to post" (John, QR); "not getting answers" (Anna, QR); and "going round in circles" (Marta, QR). In an interview, Chloe describes in great detail the "many hurdles and hoops [she had] to jump through" to access support, which are summarised in Figure 5.1, and which are especially concerning because she already felt she was "at breaking point" prior to her initial contact with mental health care services.

Chloe's experience is fairly typical in terms of the steps that are taken when help-seeking, that is, initial assessment, followed by a period of monitoring, and then a follow-up appointment. It is usually at this stage that people are offered medication and/or therapeutic treatments, with the latter often requiring further navigation through mental health services. There is often what feels like an endless cycle of "reaching out" with little resolution, being re-directed to other services or being "left to deal with it on your own" (Chloe, IR). Services

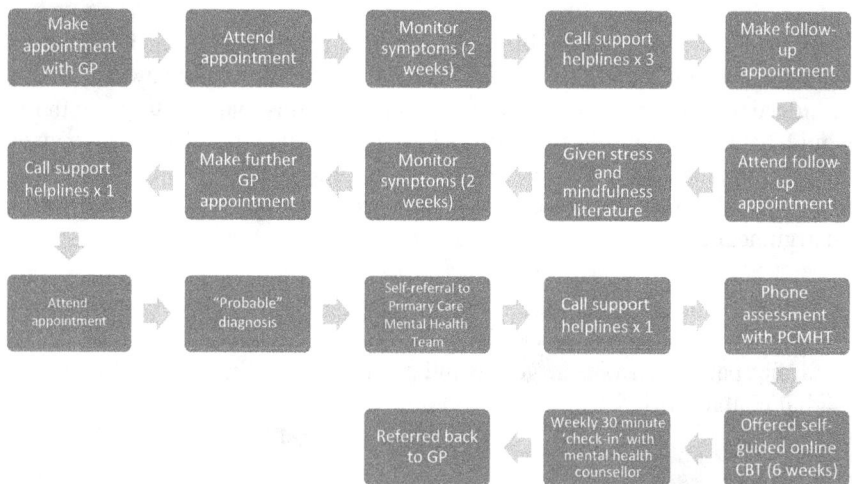

Figure 5.1 Flow chart depicting Chloe's journey of seeking a diagnosis and accessing mental healthcare services

Note: This diagram is inspired by Burgess Walsh (2023), who depicts a similar "pin-balling" between services in their diagnosis and help-seeking journey.

such as Breathing Space[5] are used as "stop gaps" between formal appointments with her General Practitioner[6] (GP) and other services when she was feeling overwhelmed or at risk of "hurting myself" (Chloe, IR). Self-referral to formal services, without the intervention of a GP, is repeatedly raised as an issue and concern in the diagnostic process. In practice, it aims to provide an "alternative entry point" to care, with the additional benefit of "help[ing] to reduce the impact of medicalisation" (Brown *et al.*, 2010). However, the face-to-face and telephone interactions involved in help-seeking and subsequent (often unexpected) self-referral processes are particularly problematic for people experiencing social anxiety: "you get yourself to the point of making an appointment, going to the appointment, talking to the doctor and THEN they tell you to refer yourself!" (Chloe, IR). One author notes similar "rounds" of asking for help and the "typically tough process" of trying to articulate emotional pain and distress and navigate a "minefield of lonely assessments and repeated conversations" only to be "sent away" and left to deal with another part of the system "on my own" (Burgess Walsh 2023, p. 7).

Affirmative experiences of diagnosis

There is social authority exercised by receiving a formal diagnosis, one that offers a certain narrative through which the "uncontrollable symptoms", "strange behaviours" and "irrational thought patterns" (Dean, QR) associated with social anxiety can be interpreted and redefined as illness:

> I am relieved that the problem has been recognised officially. It is important to me that I was diagnosed by the NHS that makes it seem more real and that I am not imagining or exaggerating it. Some people do not understand social anxiety and think it is the same as being a bit shy and that you just need to get over it. I find it difficult to tell people about SA so the official diagnosis helps me recognise it is a genuine problem and gives me confidence to refer to it if necessary.
>
> (Cara, QR)

For Cara, it is important to have her social anxiety officially recognised as it legitimises her experiences as a genuine illness, giving her permission to be ill (Nettleton, 2006). The theme of permission in relation to formal diagnosis is evident throughout participants' responses. Without one, people are afraid of being perceived as "faking it", "a failure", "attention seeking", "wasting time" and "lazy". Mark (QR) was overall ambivalent about having a diagnosis but noted that he sought one "not so much for myself, but for my family to understand I wasn't well and to help them understand why I was struggling so much". As Dumit notes, there is an "intense interplay between diagnosis and legitimacy: without a diagnosis and other forms of acceptance into the medical system, sufferers are at risk of being denied social recognition of their very suffering and accused of simply faking it" (2006, p. 578). In many cases, people find utility and intelligibility in diagnosis precisely for that reason, as a wel-come explanation for perceived "social failings" such as: "having no friends and being scared to talk to people" (Mark, QR); "coming across as rude or obnoxious" (Sam, QR); "why I can't connect with other people" (Dean, QR); "not making eye contact"; and a host symptoms including "chronic blushing, stammering, feeling awkward with strangers or public speaking, sweating, intense anxiety with new people especially attractive ones of the opposite sex, inability to think clearly, inaudible weak voice, twitching, and intense para-noia!" (Ross, QR). It also provides affirmation that: "I am not a weirdo or abnormal" (Marta, QR); "I am not crazy!" (Ross, QR); "not a coward" (Dean, QR); "it's not just me being pathetic" (Tom, QR); and validating that people are not *just* "painfully shy" and needing "to come out of my shell a bit more" (Clare, QR). Claire also added that her diagnosis:

> changed my life, it made me so happy to know I wasn't a freak and made me realise that it's a part of me but it's something I can control, not the other way around. I realised I was ill and I knew something was wrong and I was desperate for an answer and now I know it's made me so much happier to realise I'm going to be okay.

There is certainly interpretative value in the resources offered by biomedical models for describing and making sense of experience, and yet throughout these examples, there remains an unfortunate and evident tension between medical and what might be termed "moral" discourses. Diagnosis, as an objec-tive medical status, is perceived as "a more morally neutral vehicle for com-municating" mental and emotional distress (Buchman *et al.*, 2013, p. 74), there being a pervasive the sense that without a diagnosis, specifically one operating within a biomedical framing, social anxiety amounts to nothing more than a personal – indeed, "moral" – failing.

Kathryn's (IR) story particularly highlights how the explanatory power of the biomedical model is enacted through diagnostic categories:

> It took a long time for me to be diagnosed by a professional. This was very unhelpful because it made me feel like there was something wrong with me but it wasn't serious enough to be classified. However, my anxi-ety was significantly impacting my life and I didn't feel like that was being taken seriously. It was important to get a diagnosis because I didn't know which thoughts belonged to me and which were my anxious thoughts. Because I hadn't been through any trauma I was ashamed of my anxiety because I felt like it wasn't justified but the diagnosis made me feel better because it was my brain chemistry that wasn't quite right, rather than me as a person.

Kathryn's social anxiety had become all-consuming, exacerbated by both the length of time that she waited for a diagnosis and the uncertainty of whether what she was going through was even "diagnosable". Her experiences are closely tied to the idea that mental and emotional distress are a consequence of a "chemical imbalance" or a "fault in the brain's neurotransmitters" subsequently altering how her brain functions and materialising in her anxious thoughts and actions. Through diagnosis, she enacts a separation between "me" ("as a person") and "not-me" ("her anxious thoughts") through which her social anxiety is almost "written out" of her sense of who she is. It is not Kathryn who acts, but her illness. Diagnosis has an explanatory function that not only provides justification for her experiences but also absolves her from any feelings of shame or guilt. It also likely serves as a therapeutic function, one where she is not defined by her illness (Fekete, 2004).

The idea that brain chemistry is a causative rather than mediating factor is a dominant cultural narrative that has been "deeply implanted in the public psyche" (Ang, Horowitz and Moncrieff, 2022, p. 7).[7] The assessment of the more positive associations with formal diagnosis offered here suggests limitations to a more critical stance, one that might categorise all biomedical accounts as "epistemically harmful" or "unjust", but my intention has still been to offer some critical reflections on how biomedical, and more recent neurochemical, discourses are absorbed and enacted in the anxious experience. Such reflections, tugging out for a closer inspection of the criticality of participants themselves, can now be amplified.

Negative encounters

While some participants found validation and a sense of empowerment in their formal diagnosis, others did not want to be labelled with a "disorder" or "mental illness" in order to have access to necessary therapies and support. Instead, they search for more person-centred and holistic approaches that "recognise me as a person, with a history, and all the shit that entails" (Marcie, QR). Marcie also noted that diagnosis and by extension the medical model marked her "experiences as abnormal [...] in need of fixing", and yet, "the only thing they could offer me was meds that I absolutely refused bc it just feels like a plaster. It's not actually getting.to.the.root.of.it.all[8]!" Sean experienced a similar scenario:

> I went to the doctor's and tried to describe what I was feeling but I was so nervous I could only focus on how ridiculous I sounded. I felt like I wasn't being taken seriously. The doctor was really dismissive. After a few minutes he interrupted me and said, 'sounds like mild social anxiety, take these', and handed me a prescription for anti-depressants and that was it.
>
> (Sean, IR)

Hall (1996) argues that the diagnostic process for people with mental health problems under the medical model serves to undermine the individual. Participants are often required to self-report the frequency of anxiety and/or depression and the likelihood of avoidant behaviour over a two-week period. While this is arguably time and cost-efficient, since on average, it takes 8.4 minutes to diagnose the most common "mental disorders" in primary care (Jackson et al., 2001), it focuses narrowly on problems defined by clinical and biomedical frameworks resulting in "a contrived and sanctioned dehumanisation of the individual" (Hall, 1996, p. 17). The reductive and mechanistic approach in the diagnostic encounter can often have a negative impact on the individual, leaving them feeling dismissed. These factors influenced Sarah's experience of formal diagnosis following many years of self-diagnosing:

> I was in and out in 5 minutes. I'd filled out a form in the waiting room, the doctor took one look at it, put it to one side and wrote me a prescription for citalopram[9] and beta-blockers.
> L: How did that make you feel?
> S: I was kind of in shock because, even though it confirmed what I already knew, I was looking for help [and] information. Maybe even support?! I wanted someone to help me and she didn't really engage me once, didn't ask me any personal questions or nothing. I've had more in-depth appointments over a throat infection to be honest.

The focus on, and treatment of, physiological symptoms follow the principal diagnostic framework of the "disease model" (Hall, 1996; Stravynski, 2007). The lack of time and care spent on the individual's personal, familial and interpersonal history, let alone on or the daily implications of their experiences during the diagnosis of social anxiety (and mental health more generally), is emblematic of this approach. For others, the process of obtaining a formal diagnosis is "fraught [and] tedious" (Jack, QR) and "an absolute nightmare" (Lucy QR). John (QR) feels like he was "kinda forced" into a formal diagnosis, requiring it to be able to access accommodations at university that he had previously received at college without one: "I didn't want one [a diagnosis] but they [University Disability Services] refused ALL accommodations without one so really I had no choice." John's understandings of his social anxiety are couched in the idea that it is a product of "certain life events" that dominant models fail to grasp or sufficiently address. He also notes the limitations of short-term and superficial treatment such as medications and cognitive behavioural therapies, ones that he says are like "putting a plaster on stab wound". This is a general criticism of the limited treatment options available for those with social anxiety. Yet, in requiring a formal diagnosis, John is forced to align his experiences with a particular understanding of social anxiety that renders it simplistically diagnosable and treatable, one that does not "sit well with me". He continues:

> I do get it.
>   It [needing a formal diagnosis] makes sense otherwise anyone can just say anything they want 'n' get adjustments, extra time for exams 'n' all that but the red tape, hurdles 'n' stuff I had to jump [through] at both

ends [the doctor and the university] ["being passed from pillar to post" as he mentions earlier] were bloody exhausting btw.[10]

It caused so much grief I didn't need. I was just starting uni, being away from home 'n' that. It was total nightmare.

> Louise: Did it all work out though?
> Mark: Haha no, no' really. It took more work trying to get out of doing the work that just doing it!
> JK![11] I really wanted to do well in uni.
> I got the diagnosis eventually but it was about halfway through 2nd semester before they [the university] "approved" anything but by that point I was absolutely strung out[12] man, failed my first year and just dropped out.
> A total waste of time and energy all round really!

In this sense, the diagnosis was largely an administrative process to enable access to accommodations, but not an easy one to navigate both unexpectedly and at an already fraught time in John's life. However, the longer-term impacts of diagnosis for temporary accommodations at a particular time in a young person's life should be recognised, about which John says:

> It's not so bad [now] but it [the process of getting the diagnosis] really fucked me up.
> I was in an erratic place, not wanting the diagnosis, really struggling and not getting help so trying to get the diagnosis.
> It doesn't affect me so much now. Made my peace with it.
> Mostly haha.
> If I think about it too much it pisses me right off though.
> I had to eh, I've never actually put this into words, but aye[13] I'm ragin' about it, that I went through all that, like them assessing if I was "ill enough", and gave that part of my identity away for them [doctor's and university services] to …. fail to support me, I guess.

John's self-diagnosis, and validation of that diagnosis through college, hinged on the personal meanings for him as related to past life experiences. Receiving a formal diagnosis, one necessitated by his university, overlaid a particular kind of narrative that conflicted with John's self-narrative, which ultimately led to a reduced sense of (his own) agency, and further feelings of disempowerment and alienation.

Medical and therapeutic spaces

Ruga (2008) argues that the GP surgery[14] or primary care environment is comprised of three distinct environments: physical, social and generative. Physical space comprises aspects of the natural and built environment and the sites and spaces therein, including waiting rooms and doctors' offices. Social space is actively produced through interactions with others in these spaces and the properties of the space itself. The primary care environment is also conceived of as a "generative space", space one that "encourages, supports, and reinforces improvements to health and wellbeing" and is, by extension, "life-enhancing" (Ruga, 2008, 465). This concept relates to that of the "healing environment" and "evidence-based design" concerned with a more holistic understanding of how the physical environment and social space interact and condition one another. The physical and social dimensions of the surgery can also influence the doctor-patient consultation, the decision-making process within it, diagnostic effectiveness and response to treatment (Rapport, Doel and Elwyn, 2007). Previous research in the geographies of health and illness has shown that people with epilepsy (Smith, 2013) and diabetes (Lucherini, 2016) overwhelmingly feel safe in their GP surgery due, in part, to the proximity of trained and knowledgeable healthcare staff in the event of an epileptic or diabetic episode, but the same cannot necessarily be said for people experiencing social anxiety.

Physical locations can embody therapeutic qualities that harbour restorative, renewing and healing properties (Williams, 2017), but spaces intended to direct and assist in the treatment and care of people with mental health problems are not always experienced in this way and can become sources of stress and anxiety (Curtis, 2016). Georgia (IR) discusses how the physical design and organisation of her newly refurbished surgery affects her experience in the space:

> The surgery got renovated recently and the building itself makes me really anxious now. It's fucking awful. I went recently and had to go outside to calm down. By the time I came back in I'd missed my appointment and the doctor couldn't see me. [...]
>
> [The building] is a big square block. Inside the ceilings are low and corridors are long. The waiting rooms are these narrow off-shoots off the main corridors with two rows of chairs that face each other, so you're face-to-face with a stranger while you wait [and] there's absolutely no airflow, it's always swelterin'! [...] Even the colours make it sterile and clinic-y.
>
> [Before] it was kind of welcoming, a nice wee sandstone building that had some character about it. [...]
>
> They did install this wee computer to check-in for your appointment, so you don't need to speak to anyone. You just put your name and date of birth in and it tells you what doctor you're seeing and what floor and waiting room to go to. That's quite good but the rest is pretty dire.
>
> (Georgia, IR)

Despite new technology that helps Georgia to navigate the surgery space and avoid anxiety-provoking interactions with reception staff, the overall design and organisation of the building cause an unbearable sense of unease and discomfort, not least because of being confined alongside the bodies and gazes of "strangers". Recognising the difficulties that individuals experience in simply making and attending GP appointments, her existing anxieties are further heightened by entering into a known yet now unfamiliar space. The organisation of the space, with its sterile conditions and narrow spaces, prompts a negative reaction, resulting in an uncanny sense of uncertainty that leaves Georgia feeling simultaneously exposed and confined. While relations to space can shift over time as illness progresses or mobility decreases (Dyck, 1995; Crooks, 2010), the jarring transformation of an once reassuring space impacts negatively on Georgia's overall experience. Albrecht et al. (2007) coined the term "solastalgia" to explore the implications of negatively perceived or experienced changes in the environment on health and wellbeing. Although originally applied with reference to the psychological impacts of environmental change, the term has been adopted by geographers to explore the emotional reactions to changes in psychiatric hospital spaces (Wood *et al.*, 2015) demonstrating that what may be an increasingly efficient use of space for one person can cause distress for another. Georgia reflects with some nostalgia on the warmth and "character" of the original surgery, set in stark contrast to the sterile reality and modern design of the new facility. Familiarity with and attachment to place helps to establish a strong feeling of security, one that operates as a foundation from which a person can begin to grapple with and open up about distressing and emotional experiences. The shift in meaning attached to the space not only destabilises Georgia's sense of attachment but also has consequences for her overall health and wellbeing to the extent that she even missed a crucial appointment with her doctor. Lisa describes a similar experience between her first and most recent encounter with her university's Counselling and Psychological Services:

Lisa:	They renovated the building and designed this awful 'functional and efficient' space.
Louise:	Awful how?
Lisa:	It has a very white, minimal and clinical design now. The offices you go to for your initial assessment and appointments are horrible white cubicles all lined up next to each other.
	No windows!
	But the walls aren't even solid walls! They're this grey-white frosted panel. I could sort of see faint shadows from the rooms on either side and hear lots of noise, muffled voices and footsteps. It felt like there was no privacy.
	If I can hear them they can hear me sort of thing.

(Lisa, IR)

I was curious whether this had an impact on the initial assessment and the subsequent therapeutic sessions, to which she responded:

Hmm. You know wat? I've never actually thought about it in that way but yes.

I was *very* erm …

Withdrawn and hesitant, I guess, like, not able to open up cuz I was so aware of the other voices on either side and noises of people [such as] doors opening, chairs shuffling that kind of thing.

I didn't feel safe.

Exposed.

(Lisa, IR)

Unfortunately, the material features of the new design – "pods" intended to make better use of the space and frosted glass, typically intended to allow natural light to flow while retaining privacy – embody elements precisely at the heart of the anxious experience: the presence of others and of being seen or heard by them. Despite affording a certain level of privacy, the opacity still symbolises transparency and openness, providing visibility without clarity, and contributing to the feeling of being under surveillance.

Comparing the design and layout of the room where she had previously received her therapy sessions, she says:

It was nothing fancy. There was an old fireplace in the room, two mismatched armchairs and a small coffee table with some tissues on it and this little frog ornament LOL![15] But it felt cosy, sort of like my gran's house!

(Lisa, IR)

Similar to Georgia's experience, the original furnishings and organisation of the old therapy room are that of a more homely environment, one that evokes a feeling of nostalgia in Lisa as she recalls the similarities to her gran's home – a space that embodies safety and comfort for her. She describes an environment that contains the fixings of a supportive and therapeutic space, one that anticipates difficult moments (in a simple box of tissues) but also provides sensory comforts, an atmospheric calm, as well as other things to focus on (the ornament). The consequence of this is that she "never went back" (Lisa, IR) precisely because the material and personal sense of comfort afforded by the old space was lost altogether in the new one. Arguably, changes in the environment changed the nature of the therapeutic interaction itself, what was once a contained space was now one of exposure.

The contrasts – and implications – drawn here precisely mirror the broader arguments made by Högström and Philo (2023) concerning the vital geographies of mental healthcare, albeit their focus is on institutional spaces and what may be gained and lost by older and newer facilities. Offering critical reflections on the affordances of light and darkness in institutional design, they note the depth, atmospheres and senses of place lost to those now "*too* clinically ordered, clean [and] partitioned" in the name of progressive modernisation (2023, p. 332). The design of the physical, social and symbolic dimensions of therapeutic spaces can promote a sense of order, efficiency and wellbeing

(Gesler *et al.*, 2004), but those dimensions may indeed run counter to one another, with the negative features of one perhaps cancelling out the positive features of the other. While the changes implemented may have been an efficient use of space in order to accommodate growing numbers of students seeking mental healthcare and support, they succeeded in creating a highly clinical, depersonalised, even sterile atmosphere that failed to foster any sense of safety or means to promote Lisa's wellbeing.

Concluding remarks

This chapter has explored how people make sense of their experiences with social anxiety through practices of diagnosis, self-diagnosis and help-seeking. Addressing the practices of, and processes involved in, self-diagnosis specifically highlights the numerous perceptual, practical, structural and geographical barriers that people face, not only in obtaining a formal diagnosis, but in being able to access crucial therapies that may alleviate or help them navigate the intensities of their anxious distress. It then addressed what is involved for a person seeking formal diagnosis and the utility or futility of this process. While adopting an overall critical stance on the expanding scope of psychiatric diagnosis and its capacities for shaping anxious selves, bodies and experiences, this chapter has been conscious of the utility many people find in being able to name and "get a hold of" experiences of social anxiety and its associated distress that, quite frankly, rips through their social worlds. As a result, many play an active part in the medicalisation of their anxious distress, which ultimately prevents them from framing their experience through any lens other than that of the biomedical and/or neurochemical. Finally, the chapter has addressed the spaces involved in diagnosis and treatment namely doctors' surgeries and therapists' offices, to disclose, as much of this book will, how much social anxiety is entangled with a variety of social and spatial environments. The remaining chapters seek to offer more nuanced ways of understanding what lies at the heart of the anxious experience, not in search of some root or tangible cause, but rather for the ways in which it disrupts and intersects with the very ordinary routines and practices of everyday life.

Notes

1 Jutel (2009) also notes that diagnosis provides access to financial coverage; however, this is less of a concern in the UK with a publicly funded healthcare system. Healthcare is a devolved matter across the UK but payment elements exist, for example, in Scotland, Wales and Northern Ireland NHS prescriptions are free of charge whereas, in England, NHS patients have to pay prescription charges (with some exemptions).
2 Kirsty was the youngest participant at 16 years old.
3 Excessive health-related internet searches to alleviate health worries ("hypochondria" or "health anxiety") lead to further fear, distress and concern for one's health (Starcevic and Berle, 2013, p. 205).
4 Shorthand for "because".

5 Breathing Space is a telephone and webchat service delivered by NHS Scotland for those requiring immediate support for low mood, depression or anxiety.
6 Family doctor or primary care physician.
7 The "chemical imbalance theory" of mental distress is part of a much broader debate, with a wide-ranging number of actors, that space does not allow me to unpack in suitable depth here. Briefly, it is based on the theory that abnormalities in the brain structure cause mental illness, one which justified the use of anti-depressants and other psychotropics in treatment (see Ang et al. 2022 for a useful review on the historical contexts and debates).
8 The series of full stops between each word creates a pause, adds impact and signals overall frustration.
9 A brand of anti-depressants.
10 By the way.
11 Just kidding.
12 Meaning physically and emotionally exhausted.
13 Aye means yes.
14 Doctor's surgery here refers to the primary care environment in the UK, that is, doctor's office, not surgical practice.
15 Laugh out loud.

References

Albrecht, G. et al. (2007) 'Solastalgia: The distress caused by environmental change', *Australasian Psychiatry*, 15(1_suppl), pp. S95–S98. https://doi.org/10.1080/10398560701701288

Ang, B., Horowitz, M., and Moncrieff, J. (2022) 'Is the chemical imbalance an "urban legend"? An exploration of the status of the serotonin theory of depression in the scientific literature', *SSM - Mental Health*, 2, p. 100098. https://doi.org/10.1016/j.ssmmh.2022.100098

Blaxter, M. (1978) 'Diagnosis as category and process: The case of alcoholism', *Social Science & Medicine. Part A: Medical Psychology & Medical Sociology*, 12, pp. 9–17. https://doi.org/10.1016/0271-7123(78)90017-2

Boyd, D., Ryan, J. and Leavitt, A. (2011) 'Pro-self-harm and the visibility of youth-generated problematic content', *I/S: A Journal of Law and Policy for the Information Society*, 7, p. 1.

Brown, J.S. et al. (2010) 'Can a self-referral system help improve access to psychological treatments?', *The British Journal of General Practice*, 60(574), pp. 365–371. https://doi.org/10.3399/bjgp10X501877

Buchman, D.Z. et al. (2013) 'Neurobiological narratives: Experiences of mood disorder through the lens of neuroimaging', *Sociology of Health & Illness*, 35(1), pp. 66–81. https://doi.org/10.1111/j.1467-9566.2012.01478.x

Burgess Walsh, M. (2023) 'The vicious circle of reaching out and asking for help – A mental health patient's perspective', *Ethics and Social Welfare*, pp. 1–9. https://doi.org/10.1080/17496535.2023.2201990

Callard, F. (2014) 'Psychiatric diagnosis: The indispensability of ambivalence', *Journal of Medical Ethics*, 40(8), pp. 526–530. https://doi.org/10.1136/medethics-2013-101763

Campbell, R. and Longhurst, R. (2013) 'Obsessive–compulsive disorder (OCD): Gendered metaphors, blogs and online forums', *New Zealand Geographer*, 69(2), pp. 83–93. https://doi.org/10.1111/nzg.12011

Charlton, B.G. (2005) 'Self-management of psychiatric symptoms using over-the-counter (OTC) psychopharmacology: The S-DTM therapeutic model--Self-diagnosis, self-treatment, self-monitoring', *Medical Hypotheses*, 65(5), pp. 823–828. https://doi.org/10.1016/j.mehy.2005.07.013

Chen, T. et al. (2023) 'Diagnosing attention-deficit hyperactivity disorder (ADHD) using artificial intelligence: A clinical study in the UK', *Frontiers in Psychiatry*, 14. pp. 1–13, https://doi.org/10.3389/fp-syt.2023.1164433

Crooks, V.A. (2010) 'Women's changing experiences of the home and life inside it after becoming chronically ill,' in Chouinard, V., Hall, E., and Wilton, R. (eds.) *Towards Enabling Geographies: 'Disabled' Bodies and Minds in Society and Space*. London: Ashgate Publishing, pp. 45–62.

Curtis, S. (2016) *Space, Place and Mental Health*. 1st edition. London: Routledge.

Davidson, J. and Parr, H. (2010) 'Enabling cultures of dis/order online', in Chouinard, V., Hall, E., and Wilton, R., (eds.) *Towards Enabling Geographies: 'Disabled' Bodies and Minds in Society and Space*. London: Ashgate Publishing. pp. 63–84.

Dumit, J. (2006) 'Illnesses you have to fight to get: Facts as forces in uncertain, emergent illnesses', *Social Science & Medicine*, 62(3), pp. 577–590. https://doi.org/10.1016/j.socscimed.2005.06.018

Dyck, I. (1995) 'Hidden geographies: The changing lifeworlds of women with multiple sclerosis', *Social Science & Medicine*, 40(3), pp. 307–320. https://doi.org/10.1016/0277-9536(94)E0091-6

Ebeling, M. (2011) '"Get with the program!": Pharmaceutical marketing, symptom checklists and self-diagnosis', *Social Science & Medicine*, 73(6), pp. 825–832. https://doi.org/10.1016/j.socscimed.2011.05.054

Edge, D. and MacKian, S.C. (2010) 'Ethnicity and mental health encounters in primary care: Help-seeking and help-giving for perinatal depression among Black Caribbean women in the UK', *Ethnicity & Health*, 15(1), pp. 93–111. https://doi.org/10.1080/13557850903418836

Fekete, D.J. (2004) 'How I quit being a "mental patient" and became a whole person with a neurochemical imbalance: Conceptual and functional recovery from a psychotic episode', *Psychiatric Rehabilitation Journal*, 28(2), pp. 189–194. https://doi.org/10.2975/28.2004.189.194

Fox, N.J., Ward, K.J., and O'Rourke, A.J. (2005a) 'Pro-anorexia, weight-loss drugs and the internet: An "anti-recovery" explanatory model of anorexia', *Sociology of Health & Illness*, 27(7), pp. 944–971. https://doi.org/10.1111/j.1467-9566.2005.00465.x

Fox, N.J., Ward, K.J. and O'Rourke, A.J. (2005b) 'The "expert patient": Empowerment or medical dominance? The case of weight loss, pharmaceutical drugs and the Internet', *Social Science & Medicine*, 60(6), pp. 1299–1309. https://doi.org/10.1016/j.socscimed.2004.07.005

Gesler, W. et al. (2004) 'Therapy by design: Evaluating the UK hospital building program', *Health & Place*, 10(2), pp. 117–128. https://doi.org/10.1016/S1353-8292(03)00052-2

Giles, D.C. and Newbold, J. (2011) 'Self- and other-diagnosis in user-led mental health online communities', *Qualitative Health Research*, 21(3), pp. 419–428. https://doi.org/10.1177/1049732310381388

Hall, B.A. (1996) 'The psychiatric model: a critical analysis of its undermining effects on nursing in chronic mental illness', *Advances in Nursing Science*, 18, pp. 16–26.

Högström, E. and Philo, C. (2023) '"Let there be light" or life in the dark? Vital geographies of mental healthcare', *Social Science & Medicine*, 333, p. 116137. https://doi.org/10.1016/j.socscimed.2023.116137

Jackson, J.L., Houston, J.S., Hanling, S.R., Terhaar, K.A. and Yun, J.S. (2001) 'Clinical predictors of mental disorders among medical outpatients', *Archives of Internal Medicine*, 161(6), pp. 875–879. https://doi.org/10.1001/archinte.161.6.875

Jutel, A. (2009) 'Sociology of diagnosis: A preliminary review', *Sociology of Health & Illness*, 31(2), pp. 278–299. https://doi.org/10.1111/j.1467-9566.2008.01152.x

Jutel, A. (2010) 'Self-diagnosis: A discursive systematic review of the medical literature', *Journal of Participatory Medicine*, 2(8), pp. 1–13.

Jutel, A. and Nettleton, S. (2011) 'Towards a sociology of diagnosis: Reflections and opportunities', *Social Science & Medicine*, 73(6), pp. 793–800. https://doi.org/10.1016/j.socscimed.2011.07.014

Leigh, E., Chiu, K., and Ballard, E.D. (2023) 'Social anxiety and suicidality in youth: A systematic review and meta-analysis', *Research on Child and Adolescent Psychopathology*, 51(4), pp. 441–454. https://doi.org/10.1007/s10802-022-00996-0

Lewis, L.F. (2017) 'A mixed methods study of barriers to formal diagnosis of autism spectrum disorder in adults', *Journal of Autism and Developmental /Disorders*, 47(8), pp. 2410–2424. https://doi.org/10.1007/s10803-017-3168-3

Lucherini, M. (2016) 'Performing diabetes: Surveillance and self-management', *Surveillance & Society*, 14(2), pp. 259–276. https://doi.org/10.24908/ss.v14i2.5996

Lupton, D. and Jutel, A. (2015) '"It's like having a physician in your pocket!" A critical analysis of self-diagnosis smartphone apps', *Social Science & Medicine*, 133, pp. 128–135. https://doi.org/10.1016/j.socscimed.2015.04.004

Mackian, S. (2002) 'A Review of Health Seeking Behaviour: Problems and Prospects', *Health Systems Development. University of Manchester, Manchester, UK.* [Preprint].

Mackintosh, N. et al. (2020) 'Online resources and apps to aid self-diagnosis and help seeking in the perinatal period: A descriptive survey of women's experiences', *Midwifery*, 90, p. 102803. https://doi.org/10.1016/j.midw.2020.102803

Nettleton, S. (2006) '"I just want permission to be ill": Towards a sociology of medically unexplained symptoms', *Social Science & Medicine*, 62(5), pp. 1167–1178. https://doi.org/10.1016/j.socscimed.2005.07.030

Nettleton, S. and Burrows, R. (2003) 'E-scaped medicine? Information, reflexivity and health', *Critical Social Policy*, 23(2), pp. 165–185. https://doi.org/10.1177/0261018303023002003

NICE (2013) Social anxiety disorder: Recognition, assessment and treatment. *Clinical Guideline*, 159 (No. 159).

Olfson, M. et al. (2000) 'Barriers to the treatment of social anxiety', *American Journal of Psychiatry*, 157(4), pp. 521–527. https://doi.org/10.1176/appi.ajp.157.4.521

Parr, H. (2002) 'New body-geographies: The embodied spaces of health and medical information on the internet', *Environment and Planning D: Society and Space*, 20(1), pp. 73–95. https://doi.org/10.1068/d41j

Parr, H. and Philo, C. (2003) 'Rural mental health and social geographies of caring', *Social & Cultural Geography*, 4(4), pp. 471–488. https://doi.org/10.1080/1464936032000137911

Prior, L. (2003) 'Belief, knowledge and expertise: The emergence of the lay expert in medical sociology', *Sociology of Health & Illness*, 25(3), pp. 41–57. https://doi.org/10.1111/1467-9566.00339

Rapport, F. A., Doel, M. and Elwyn, G. (2007) 'Snapshots and snippets: General practitioners' reflections on professional space', *Health & Place*, 13(2), pp. 532–544. https://doi.org/10.1016/j.healthplace.2006.07.005

Rose, N. (2003) 'Neurochemical selves', *Society*, 41(1), pp. 46–59. https://doi.org/10.1007/BF02688204

Rose, N. (2006) 'Disorders without borders? The expanding scope of psychiatric practice', *Biosocieties*, 1, pp. 465–484. https://doi.org/10.1017/S1745855206004078

Rosenberg, C.E. (2002) 'The tyranny of diagnosis: Specific entities and individual experience', *The Milbank Quarterly*, 80(2), pp. 237–260. https://doi.org/10.1111/1468-0009.t01-1-00003

Ross Arguedas, A.A. (2022) 'Diagnosis as subculture: Subversions of health and medical knowledges in the orthorexia recovery community on Instagram', *Qualitative Sociology*, 45(3), pp. 327–351. https://doi.org/10.1007/s11133-022-09518-2

Ruga, W. (2008) 'Your general practice environment can improve your community's health', *The British Journal of General Practice*, 58(552), pp. 460–462. https://doi.org/10.3399/bjgp08X302961

Smith, N.D. (2013) *The everyday social geographies of living with epilepsy*. PhD. University of Glasgow. https://eleanor.lib.gla.ac.uk/record=b3004343 (Accessed: 26 May 2023).

Stanghellini, G. (2004) 'The puzzle of the psychiatric interview', *Journal of Phenomenological Psychology*, 35(2), pp. 173–195. https://doi.org/10.1163/1569162042652191

Starcevic, V. and Berle, D. (2013) 'Cyberchondria: Towards a better understanding of excessive health-related Internet use', *Expert Review of Neurotherapeutics*, 13(2), pp. 205–213. https://doi.org/10.1586/ern.12.162

Stravynski, A. (2007). *Fearing Others: The Nature and Treatment of Social Phobia*. Cambridge University Press.

Tucker, I.M. and Lavis, A. (2019) 'Temporalities of mental distress: Digital immediacy and the meaning of "crisis" in online support', *Sociology of Health & Illness*, 41(S1), pp. 132–146. https://doi.org/10.1111/1467-9566.12943

Williams, A. (2017) *Therapeutic Landscapes*. London: Routledge.

Wood, V.J. et al. (2015) '"Therapeutic landscapes" and the importance of nostalgia, solastalgia, salvage and abandonment for psychiatric hospital design', *Health & Place*, 33, pp. 83–89. https://doi.org/10.1016/j.healthplace.2015.02.010

6 Spatialities of anxious experience I

Home and workplaces

Introduction

Chapters 6 and 7 are written as a couplet to provide an in-depth exploration of the social and spatial contingencies of living with social anxiety in order to map its disrupted and disruptive geographies. Where this chapter attends to home and work, spaces inherently related to health and wellbeing in both material and psychosocial capacities, the next, Chapter 7, builds a more expansive geography of public spaces and mobilities that permeates the anxious experience, while simultaneously digging deeper into the relational and embodied encounters occurring across such sites. The institutional entanglements of home and work have long been a focus in the geographies of mental health, which have been attentive to the wide range of therapies and pathways towards "recovery" for individuals in community and acute mental healthcare settings (Parr, Philo and Burns, 2003; Philo, Parr and Burns, 2005). These spaces are addressed together as how people experience, are supported through and potentially "recover" from mental and emotional distress, illness and/or trauma is particularly wrapped up in the environments that they typically inhabit for the longest periods of time, both daily and across a life-course.

First, this chapter attends to the spaces of home as everyday sources of distress through themes of fragmented spaces, domestic routines and anticipatory objects. It does so in recognition that the daily grind of social anxiety impinges on the social, material and emotional dimensions of home. It thereby demonstrates the extent to which the experience of home, as a place separated from public life and a refuge from external anxieties, is upended by the anxious experience. It addresses home spaces and objects in order to understand how the boundaries of home are complicated, experienced and negotiated, as well as considering how the various temporalities of home, whether in the routines of daily life or through the gradual or sudden demands of home and family life, assuage or aggravate anxieties.

This chapter also focuses on the socio-spatial challenges associated with the workplace in order to grasp how employment spheres of life have been disrupted over the life course of individuals who manage (and struggle) to gain and maintain education and then employment opportunities.[1] There is a

DOI: 10.4324/9781003206880-6

focus on the everyday management and negotiation of these spaces that pays attention to interactions and performances that fuel social anxieties – for example, giving presentations or speaking to people in authority – and for my participants become increasingly fearful and disabling aspects of everyday life. Attention is additionally paid to the tensions and stigma that arise in relation to working with a (known[2]) mental health problem at this juncture between (reli)ability and recovery. Participants share detailed accounts about how their careers have been disrupted by pervasive anxieties and fears, often reflecting on personal and structural barriers – and then the psychological and physiological consequences – of trying to (re)gain and maintain meaningful participation in work-related activities. This aspect bled into further discussions in interviews about the temporal, spatial and emotional work involved in managing and negotiating everyday life with their mental health problems (Laws, 2013).

Home

Recent geographical engagements with home have evaluated the spaces, practices, relations and materialities at play in the making and unmaking of home. Traditionally, the home has prompted rather static notions as a place of unmitigated safety, one saturated with emotions and nostalgia, where traditions, values and connections instil a sense of belonging and connection, and a place that is deeply intertwined with our personal and shared identities. Dupuis and Thorns (1998, p. 29) argue that in a world frequently "experienced as threatening and uncontrollable", the home is best conceived of as a "site of constancy", one that "allows for a sense of control" and provides a "secure base around which identities can be constructed". The idea of home is negotiated and made sense of through a number of physical spaces (living room, bedroom), social relations (family, friends, visitors, neighbours) and objects within the home (telephones, windows, doors, doorbells). It is the place we leave from and the place we return to and the foundation through which many routines and rituals of personal and familial life are established. The geographies of home are overlapping and conflicting, constituted by "multiple material and imagined spaces in which different social relations are expressed, enacted and experienced" (Mclean, 2008a, p. 564). The taken-for-granted understandings of home as a "stronghold" are acutely contested and disrupted through innumerable experiences such as harassment, hate and control (Valentine, 1998; Burch, 2023), domestic violence (Warrington, 2001), austerity and precarity (Kane, 2023), and with the onset and progression of illness or disability (Moss, 1997; Dyck, 1998). In such scenarios, the home can symbolise the loss of independence and social identity and, rather than a place of anchorage, becomes a site of entrapment, confinement or even avoidance. Thus, home is better conceived of as a space that "disappoints, aggravates, neglects, confines and contradicts as much as it inspires and comforts us" (Moore, 2000, p. 213), and it is this tension that the following aims to illuminate.

Fragmented home spaces

It is perhaps unsurprising that when asked about feelings of safety associated with home, participants overwhelmingly consider their home to be a "safe" or "very safe" space. However, in unpacking what it was *about* home (its constituent spaces, relations and materialities) that made it an inherently safe place, participants reveal a much more spatially complex and contingent geography of the home than one is simply "safe" or "unsafe". For many, home is deemed a safe and secure space simply because it sits in stark contrast to the open and collective nature of everyday social and public spaces (Chapter 7). Sam (QR) describes home as a place to "hide from the world" and Olivia (QR) says her "anxiety is less active at home". Sarah (IR) notes that she does not "feel safe outside", highlighting that time and distance away from home can also become an issue: "on top of feeling like I'm drawing attention to myself [outside], the longer I'm out the worse it gets and I'm scared my anxiety will get so bad that I won't make it home." Home is deemed a safe place to return to, where the anxieties and expectations of the outside world can be "left behind":

> I feel safer here [at home] because it's my space, you know? My own little part of the world that is solely my own.
>   I live alone and have complete control over this space, who comes to visit, who I answer the door to or who I speak to. I know when I close the front door I feel safe and there's a feeling of relief that comes with that expectation disappearing.
>   I get home and these four walls are like armour.
>
> (Mia, IR)

> I go to work and come home that's my day really. [...]
>   Home is absolutely my safe haven and the place I can retreat into at the end of the day and try and bring the cycle of anxiety down a few notches [through] my evening routines and generally just trying to wind down and relax
>
> (Lauren, IR)

In experiences of agoraphobia, which are most similar to the geographies discussed herein, the boundaries of home often come to represent a "reinforcement and extension of the psycho-corporeal boundaries of the self" (Davidson, 2000, p. 35). Establishing personal territories and territorial practices within the home space often aids in regaining a sense of control over the uncontrollable, such as other people or germs (Davidson, 2000; Segrott and Doel, 2004). Mia and Lauren both live alone and home is a place that they can seek private and unseen refuge at the end of the day. A sense of safety is established by being able to retain (or regain) a more cohesive sense of self but with slightly different connotations of what that safety entails and how it is obtained for each of them. For Mia, the boundaries of home mark a clear distinction between "inside", associated with feelings of safety and security, and the world "outside" where uncertainty and social expectations are rife. She also conveys a deep sense of attachment, ownership and protection that resonates with Porteous' (1976) understanding of home as a "territorial core", that is, a foundational place through which psychological and physical security are established and maintained. The idea of home being her "own little part of the world" confers a sense of ownership that promotes both personal integrity and identity. Through the material boundaries of home, which act like "armour", and personal defences, that is, controlling who comes in, Mia creates a "stable refuge" (Porteous 1976, p. 390) from the pressures and expectations of the outside world. Lauren's idea of home as a "haven" is less "territorial" than Mia's, but rather one embodying the restorative potential of home through the familiarity of "evening routines" that are integral to her emotional wellbeing.

Outside of routines that form the "bedrock" of daily life, there is often a lack of spontaneity about leaving the house and as a result people's daily geographies are fairly restricted: "Other than going to work and doing a food shop, I really don't leave the house" (Lauren, IR).[3] A significant amount of time and energy is also invested in simply preparing to leave the home (Chapter 8). Once outside, the possibilities of meeting, seeing and hearing other people – along with the combined impact of interactions, whether a friendly greeting or sustained social activity – in social and public spaces continue to provoke intense anxieties and feelings of overwhelm (Chapter 7). As a result, people often need to "disconnect", removing themselves in order to recover from the multiple and competing demands of the social world (Moss, 1997). With this in mind, Craig (IR) notes that it is "often not worth" going outside in the first place. As a result, participants' social geography is commonly restricted to prolonged periods of homebound isolation through which home comes to occupy a more disruptive and contested position in people's everyday lives. This situation is recognised in different ways, with Lauren (IR) noting that "sometimes I just get sick of staring at the same four walls"; while Kirsty (QR) recognises that when she is at home she is "isolated and alone, which is good for the anxiety", but it is not necessarily conducive to her overall health and wellbeing. Meanwhile, Craig says that he regularly gets "cabin fever" and feels "cooped up", but even though he is "sick of being inside all the time [...] as soon as I go outside I want to come back in" (Craig, IR). Dawn (QR) also writes, "I wish I didn't have to ever leave the house. It's not that I get any actual enjoyment out of staying home a lot", and adds that she finds "it harder to go outside when I don't go out for extended periods of time". The home can become as confining and claustrophobic as it is protective and restorative, particularly for those who find the solitude of home inescapable. In recounting her experiences with agoraphobia in which she "became habituated to a contracted world", Bordo (Bordo, Klein and Silverman, 1998, p. 62) states that stepping outside acted as a momentary "inoculation" that loosened the constraints felt by her "homeboundness" just enough to enable her to find stasis and orientation again within it.

Despite the protective and therapeutic offerings of home, it can also be experienced as an everyday space of distress, leading to more spatially fragmented and constrained senses of home. The experiences in and perceptions of the home are prone to disruption from multiple factors, including the ebbs and flows of social anxiety itself. Beth (IR), who has been more or less housebound for an extended period of time, discusses how her "safe bubble" and thus where she feels able to go within and around her home (garden, street, wider neighbourhood) shifts in response to her mental health highlighting the fluctuating nature of anxious experiences:

> On days when my anxiety isn't too bad, I might be able to go into the garden for some fresh air and hope the neighbours aren't around. On really bad days, which aren't too frequent now thank god, you're lucky if I can leave my room.
> On really good days I could go a bit further and that's happening a little more now, which is good news I guess:)

Similarly, the (often unwelcome) presence and comings and goings of others within and around the home greatly colour people's anxieties. Generally, the relationships with family co-habitants are discussed positively as essential sources of support and social life, for example, a partner, siblings and older children, although this can cause relational strain and feelings of shame when people feel they are "so reliant on someone else to function in the world" (Amelia, QR) or when family members do not understand the anxiety being experienced (Chapter 7). Moreover, the presence and anticipation of others, whether that be wider family, visitors, neighbours, landlords, social workers, tradespeople or strangers, can preoccupy home life, causing significant distress that complicates any feelings of home-based safety. Bennett (2011) explores how the physical presence of others results in the young women in her research feeling "homeless" at home, sentiments echoed in this research by participants whose neighbours "watch every move I make", or whose home life is disrupted by "surprise visits" (Moira, QR), "family turning up unannounced" (Amelia, QR), or "when the kids' friends are over" (Tina, QR):

> I live at home [with parents and siblings] and there's aaaalways people around. It drives me nuts.
> My brother's girlfriend stays a lot and my aunts are always round or on the phone.
> Even our next-door neighbours are in and out
> UNannounced.
> I just really, really struggle with it. Ughhhh[4].
> If anyone is in I won't go downstairs and also don't spend that much time downstairs cos someone will just randomly appear. I'm always on edge about it. So it's safer for me to stay in my room and if people are in I just stay put […]

Mum gets so angry, especially if it's family. She just doesn't get it and thinks I'm so rude :(([5]

The presence of others often changes the temporal rhythms of being at home too, with many participants preferring night-time over day-time as there are "no expectations, no one's moving around, [it's] more peaceful" (Craig, QR):

Clare: My sleep schedule is pretty messed up. I'm awake until about 3am most nights but I love it when everyone else has gone to bed
    The street is empty, there's no noise from neighbours, family aren't roaming about the house.
    I feel like I'm truly alone.

Louise: What do you do?

C: Totally and completely relax! Lie in bed mostly but read, watch films, play video games. Just snuggle up.
    The total darkness is nice too.

A number of participants speak about keeping "night shift" patterns, being more awake and active while others are typically sleeping:

I prefer night over day. I'm definitely a night owl. During the day I am depressed and feel ashamed when I can't leave the house. At night that same feeling doesn't really weigh as heavy.
    Everything is more relaxed and quiet.

Such dissonant rhythms are typically conceived as having negative implications for health and wellbeing, such as for those working shifts or experiencing insomnia (Collier, Skitt and Cutts, 2003), and stand in stark contrast to the temporalities of those living with Seasonal Affective Disorder, who experience negative effects to shorter days, reduced light and social contact during the winter months (Bodden *et al.*, 2022). Social anxieties, although not disappearing entirely at night, especially if there is an event to anticipate the next day, are nonetheless abated in some measure by the night's lack of social contact and expectation.

Domestic routines

Two participants with children discuss how their social anxiety is caught up in the daily geographies of home life, both exacerbated and appeased by the roles and routines of domestic life. Both participants were, for the most part, housebound and highlight the various ways that the roles and responsibilities of motherhood are entangled with their social anxieties, contributing to their experiences of being housebound in both positive and negative ways. Karen, a single mother of three young children whose social anxiety began shortly after the birth of her third child, says:

I'm comfortable and safe here; it's just my own surroundings. I did go out with my sister. That was only the other week and I hadn't been out the house in like six weeks just out in the garden and stuff [pause] that's my safe place and I don't want to leave.

(Karen, IR)

Rather than a state, being "housebound" is better understood as an act of safe-keeping (Davidson, 2009) in the face of experiences of social anxiety, which Karen states have a "horrendous" impact on her day-to-day life. She experiences intense anxiety about being outside the confines of her home and equally so about interacting with people from her close-knit community who may have noticed her absence from community life, ask questions and spread gossip: "you know like, 'how come her mum does the school run?' and all that" (Karen, IR). Neighbourhoods and local communities circulating the spaces of home can be perceived as potentially dangerous places (Bankey, 1999). Examining women's experiences of social anxiety, where anxieties are articulated through certain societal discourses, norms and expectations of femininity, Masters (2021) notes that motherhood is subject to particular forms of "cultural surveillance" regarding perceived "commitment to motherhood" (Downing 2019, *as cited in* Masters 2021, p. 221). Schmied and Kearney (2018, p. 9) also discuss the maternal anxieties that emerge in relation to "good mother" ideologies, often "conflict[ing] with the reality of women's lives". Tina, who has three teenage children, discusses similar feelings of guilt in relation to home and family life: "I feel like a failure for my son and I always really wanted to be involved with school life but got knocked back a lot and it made me more anxious. So I kind of gave up". She also comments on her reliance on her children for help: "I ask my oldest children for support everyday" (Tina, QR). Masters (2021, p. 310) argues that "female socialisation", and by extension the aspects of motherhood highlighted here, "fosters feelings of inadequacy" that lie at the heart of social anxiety.

Karen has frequent and recurring panic attacks and can experience up to four panic attacks "on a good day", even within the relative security of her home. Her home is a known and predictable environment offering privacy to manage routinely unpredictable bodily experiences, where she has access to medication to control intense periods of anxiety and where she practices established domestic and daily routines:

I just keep myself busy in the house [...] I try to keep busy doing housework and just doing things, you know, like hanging out the washing and maybe sitting out the back [garden]. I'll sit out there and take my medication. I'm okay in the house [...] I can help cook their [her children's] dinner, help them do their homework, help them get dressed or ready for bed. My son, I bath him in the morning. Homework and stuff is not a problem. I just cannot take them over that front door.

(Karen, IR)

Throughout the interview, Karen speaks about wanting "to be a good mother" and how she feels "guilty", and "worried about the impact" that her health has on her children and her relationship with them. She feels it is even more important to facilitate a homely and caring environment because she is unable to play an active part in their school or extracurricular lives beyond it. Home life is punctuated by being able to do "little things" that aid in the everyday management of social anxiety or as a component part of longer-term mental health recovery. She places particular importance on roles and rituals practised within the home such as doing homework, cooking and eating together, as well as bedtime routines, and also views home as a place to prepare for "bigger things like going to GP and CPN[6] appointments" (Karen, IR) that provide a path towards better management and recovery. It is through these habitual practices that she establishes and maintains a positive sense of home and establishes more "positive" senses of self as a "good mother", remaining active through her cyclical bouts of panic and also performing as a "good patient" by remaining engaged with mental health services. Bankey[7] (1999, p. 173) argues that these health experiences and practices are "tragically self-defeating [...] reinforc[ing] the stereotypical gendered nature of the 'home' or domestic sphere, repeating patterns of oppression [and] domestic ideals that further immobilise them". Ultimately though, the home is a space where Karen feels safe and empowered, having built a stronger and more stable sense of self in the home through routines and social roles, even if gendered, standing in stark contrast to her sense of self outside of it, where she has "no control". The practices of home-making see her home spaces "re-made in more affirmative ways" (Burch, 2023, p. 13). In many ways, her home is a site of resistance that, while occasionally disrupted, is where her socio-spatial and bodily boundaries remain, for the most part, intact.

Anticipatory objects

Anticipatory objects[8] are those typical every day and unremarkable material objects that establish a particular spatiality and temporality within the home. Spatially, they are markers of gaps and potential intrusions in the carefully managed boundaries of home. Temporally, they embody an "uncertain immanence" (Leyshon, Née and Geoghegan, 2012, p. 240), an expectation, a potential exposure or encounter; a case of not "if" but "when" will the safety of home be breached by others. Material objects are not passive but active, with potentialities and capacities, and actively involved in the production and experience of social relations and space. Household materialities, including telephones, windows, "thin" walls, elevators, doors, doorbells and electronic entry systems, all embody an intimate exteriority, whereby the "outside" is felt as "inside" as always present and ever-encroaching. In experiences of epilepsy, Smith (2013, p. 192) highlights that, although home provides relative social and physical safety, compared with public spaces, in the event of a seizure, the normally inconspicuous "surfaces, textures and spaces" of the home often impose a higher risk of accident and injury. While the concern in the present study is not the risk of physical injury, everyday objects are similarly imbued with risk, that of being "seen" and "heard" by others as well as embodying the threat of interaction looming from the outside. The concept of anticipation in human geography is typically invoked in relation to particular objects and practices that "create, know and govern possible, potential or preferred futures" and "alleviate future uncertainties" (Anderson, 2007, p. 158) but anticipation is also considered in the context of an object's capacity to provoke particular "physical, social and emotional movements" (Larsen, Bøe and Topor, 2020). Participants often mention these objects in relation to their attempts to break connections with the social world beyond the home by closing curtains, turning off entry systems, and "unhooking" home telephones or having mobile phones on "silent" or "do not disturb" modes. As part of the wider materiality of home, these mundane artefacts are "caught up in the currents of the lifeworld" (Ingold, 2007, p. 1) and integral to shaping particular relationships and contexts with/in it:

> When the doorbell rings, I jump out my skin. I almost go into a panic attack. I have shortness of breath and my heartbeat races and have tons of fear about who is on the other side of the door. Most of the time I can't even bring myself to move to answer it. I get so terrified that they'll hear me and will know I'm home hiding from them. I sit there rigid, panicking, until they go away.
>
> (Eva, IR)

Valentine (1998, p. 321) discusses how "simple objects" and "everyday sounds" can radically disrupt the everyday "taken-for-grantedness" of home environments. Despite its commonplace nature, the doorbell is a signal that *someone is there*, but the unexpected and unknown *who* provokes distressing bodily and emotional reactions:

> Anxiety SPIKES if someone knocks the door, especially if I'm not expecting anyone.
>
> (Craig, QR)

> I live in a flat and have one of those wee spyhole things on the door so I can check if anyone is in the close[9] before I leave to try and avoid bumping into anyone.
>
> (Rosie, IR)

For similar reasons, telephones become a source of anxiety as an abrupt and unexpected interruption in the home. Rosie says that she routinely:

> [...] unplug[s] the phone unless I know I'm expecting a call [...]
>   my mum phones on a Saturday so I'll plug it back in on a Saturday morning.
>
> (Rosie, IR)

While disruptions like those outlined above may occur in a single moment if, for example, "someone appears at the door unexpectedly" (Olivia, QR), participants also recount having to deal with longer-term and more continuous disruptions evident throughout the course of a day or in shifting expectations between during the week and weekends (Mclean, 2008b). In his questionnaire response, Brian lists some scenarios in his home that provoke anxiety, drawing particular attention to:

> Someone at the door: buzzer[10] goes constantly during the day/week, parcel and food deliveries for neighbours, postman etc. needing [to get] in the building. [I feel] constantly on edge that they know I'm in/ignoring them/they can hear me once in the building. Night time and weekends are nice, very quiet. More relaxing.
>
> (Brian, QR)

Dupuis and Thorns (1998, p. 27) argue that the private realm of the home is also one "where tensions built up from the constant surveillance in other settings of daily life can be relieved", and for some participants, like Mia and Lauren outlined at the beginning of this chapter, that sense of relief is absolutely the case. But for others, the possibility of "surveillance" from the outside, of being seen or heard by neighbours and others, punctures the presumed "at-ease-ness" of being at home:

> Home is a weird one. Obviously I feel safe-ish here but I don't have that feeling of pure freedom, like I'm never fully relaxed. I don't even feel like I can move around freely. I hate being near the windows in case someone sees me so tend to keep the lights off at night and the blinds angled in a way where they can't see me.
>
> (Jess, IR)

> I feel like I have no privacy even at in my flat. I'm finally in my refuge but the walls are thin and my windows are level with the street so anyone passing can see inside.
>   See ME inside.
>
> (Kim, IR)

In the separation of the public and private domains of life, walls are the most obvious boundary markers, the dividing lines between inside and outside, but participants are troubled by the porosity of them, with "thin" walls inferring that being able to hear neighbours also means a risk of being heard *by* them. Although the home is experienced as "safe", windows and walls are mediating devices and signifiers of a "gap" in the protective boundaries of home. They are particular sources of intense discomfort that speak to the wider social anxieties about being visible to others, leaving the socially anxious fearfully open to potential judgement and scrutiny even when supposedly separated off from the wider world in their own domestic cocoon. As such, the seemingly private

spaces of home can be understood more as a "turbulent sea of constant negotiation rather than simply some haven for the self" (Miller, 2001, p. 4).

Housing conditions

Housing, broadly conceived, was not a specific focus of this research but it is
worth reflecting on the experiences of two tenants whose experiences highlight
some wider entanglements between social anxiety and the power dynamics,
status and security associated with rented accommodation. Jess and Jane both
discuss how the relations with landlords and other agencies provoke specific
anxieties which, in turn, impacts on their living conditions and the taken-for-
granted feelings of security and control typically associated with home
environments:

> It actually affects my living standards too. So, right now the kitchen sink
> keeps blocking when I do the dishes. I've spent a fair amount [of time
> and money] trying to fix it myself with drain cleaners and stuff but it
> hasn't worked. I wanted to try everything before bothering my landlord.
> So I did [try everything].
> Then spent hours deep cleaning the whole flat so it looks presentable
> and then couldn't bring myself to call him.
> And there's mould/damp in the bathroom but that's probably my fault
> for not opening the window or whatever.
> I don't want to bother him with sort of trivial things.
>
> (Jess, IR)

> My landlord or the letting agency do these random checks on the flat
> four times a year, so bloody excessive! I'd get one of two but four! I wish
> they'd just asked 'are there any issues?' I'd let them know but instead they
> want to come in and inspect the full flat.
> It just feels like a total invasion of my privacy and like I can't be
> trusted to live here. [...]
> From the moment they give notice to the minute they leave, for weeks,
> I'm up to 'high doh'[11]! It's awful but I just deal with it.
>
> (Jane, IR)

There is an overriding sense of surveillance that feeds into their anxious experiences but also sweeps through the "emotional fabric of home" (Bennett,
2011, p. 981). Jess, ensuring her flat is "presentable", is concerned that she may
be judged as messy, dirty or even negligent of a home that is not her "own",
while the routine "invasion" of Jane's privacy through "random" and "excessive" inspections leaves her riding waves of anticipation and anxiety throughout the year. Both situations allude to issues of social status and power
relations that are not only aggravating and disconcerting but, as Stravynski
(2014) argues, integral to the interpersonal pattern of social anxiety in and of
itself. The asymmetry in the tenant-landlord relationship and the power and

surveillance exerted result in feelings of insecurity, powerlessness and perhaps alienation from the home space (McKee, Soaita and Hoolachan, 2020). The "status" of renting also impacts both women: Jane mentions that her parents are urging her to buy a house even though she cannot afford it, which leaves her "embarrassed that I'm the only one [in her family] not on the property ladder". In this case, "renting is not held in the same esteem as home ownership" (McKee et al., 2020, p. 1480), leaving her feeling "less than" while also fuelling social comparisons and anxieties about her social "status". A similar dynamic exists for Jess in the sense that she may be bothersome to or burden on her landlord with (what is arguably necessary) property maintenance, resulting in her living in potentially unsafe and damp conditions. Finally, in "dealing with" the repeated intrusions (Jane) and going to great lengths to make sure her flat is clean and tidy (Jess), both women ensure that they are being "good tenants". Neither has had overtly negative interactions with their landlords but, overall, their home life is subject to a scrutiny which undermines their ability to feel secure and settled in their homes, aspects going some way to highlight "the lingering, sometimes intangible, often damaging presence of others" (Bennett, 2011, p. 963) in the home lives of the socially anxious.

Workspaces

There are commonplace assumptions made about people who experience "enduring mental health problems, [is] that they are unable to work unless, or until, they have recovered", where questions of willingness, reliability, ability and productivity arise (Grove et al., 2005). Employment is also viewed as a significant step in the process of recovery and social inclusion (Evans and Wilton, 2019). Beynon and Tucker (2006, p. 78) argue that "while people with ill health and disability have positive attitudes to work, their capacity to work is limited by multiple and often mutually reinforcing barriers". Previous research in this regard consistently demonstrates that "social anxiety has negative impacts on occupational functioning" (Himle *et al.*, 2014, p. 924). Individuals are likely to experience downward social mobility associated with unemployment or underemployment, coupled with a likely deterioration of workplace knowledges, skills and experiences over time that can have a significant impact on future employment prospects and overall health and wellbeing. Questionnaire respondents highlight numerous personal and structural barriers in their attempts to gain and maintain employment: "I have never been, or would ever be, able to go for an interview" (Kim, QR); or to advance within/beyond their current role due to "flatly reject[ing] any possibility of promotion" (Tina, QR). Callum (QR) captures the impact that social anxiety has had on these inter-related spheres of his life, initially on his academic attainment and then the subsequent effect on his employment opportunities:

> I managed to graduate from university but feel that I could have achieved a better degree (I got a 2:2) if I had been able to attend lectures, seminars, tutorials etc. I have had no career, just a succession of menial jobs,

because I fall apart in an interview situation. When I did work, I was unable to remain in any job for more than two years, as I would be ostracised by colleagues or become depressed because of the isolation. As time progressed, finding work became harder and harder, because my work record was so poor and because I have never had a promotion, with the result that I have not had a permanent job since 2004 and not worked at all since 2010.

(Callum, QR)

Callum's experience relays the implications of these anxieties on aspects of attendance and engagement in higher education, spelling out all-too-predictable ramifications for his subsequent career trajectory to the point where he ceased being able to do paid work at all. Many of the wider societal impacts of social anxiety are hence crystallised in Callum's experience. It was noted that people with mental health problems are often plagued by various forms of psychological distress, including low self-esteem, and restricted by a lack of "job skills (basic and specific)[...], work experience [...] and low education levels". This is particularly pertinent for people experiencing social anxiety where distress is centred around, and exacerbated by, a perceived inability to "perform" adequately across many social situations, including interview situations. Despite being in full-time employment, Sol's social anxiety has had a markedly impacted on his ability to progress in or beyond his current position: "[social anxiety] has definitely affected my career progression as I am too nervous to attend interviews/give presentations" (Sol, QR) While hampering those already in employment, the anxiety and fear can also be disabling for those who are actively looking for work. As Jo writes:

I have been looking for work for four years but I freak out whenever I get a job reply so [I] often chicken out as I can't manage the anxiety that goes with an interview. I've cancelled and rescheduled so many interviews because the anxiety is unbearable.

(Jo, QR)

Jo's anxieties, in a similar way to Callum's, greatly hamper her ability to gain employment and further experience within the workplace, reinforcing her pervasive feelings of failure and self-doubt. Long periods of unemployment are also a significant barrier to securing future employment (Grove et al., 2005), moreover, and Callum's education and work history are symptomatic of the conditions that create a vicious cycle of social exclusion and un(der)employment may arise in the life courses of the socially anxious.

Once through the workplace door with a contract or even just attending for an interview, such difficult hurdles for many living with social anxiety, matters do not necessarily get any easier. Geographers exploring "non-accommodating" and difficult-to-negotiate workplaces for people with disabilities (Wilton, 2004), chronic illness (Dyck, 1999; Dyck and Jongbloed, 2000) and mental health problems (Evans and Wilton, 2016; Martin, 2021), all highlight the barriers and tensions in accessing, maintaining and (re)negotiating workplaces with, or after the onset of, ill-health and/or disability. Similar to those experiencing chronic illness, social anxiety in the workplace can be inherently disabling despite its relative invisibility in comparison with, say, physical impairment. Despite being able to "pass as normal" (Davidson and Henderson, 2010), even if they feel painfully out of place, people experiencing social anxiety face difficulties accessing and negotiating the workplace through a subtle set of mechanisms present in the immediate social and material environment, as will now be elaborated.

As highlighted above by Jo, the hiring process is a significant barrier to gaining employment for people with social anxiety. The interview is an intensely anticipated event during which an individual's performance is assessed and scrutinised. This encounter can be extremely distressing, as Sophie (IR) and Lara (IR) both relate:

Sophie: I've had so many bad experiences and failed attempts that I can't even think about trying to look for a job at this point. The last job I applied for was over a year ago and from the moment [the interview] was scheduled it consumed my every waking thought; I couldn't sleep for worrying about it. Every day for weeks I had this feeling in the pit of my stomach that something was going to happen. Constantly playing over all the things in my head that could/would go wrong

Louise: What like?

S: Oh, like, not being able to answer questions, failing miserably, being visibly anxious, like, shaking and blushing, having a panic attack, being judged, them thinking I'm stupid or incompetent and having them staring at me, face-to-face situations are crippling and the fear of failing. All of it. It's just terrifying. Embarrassing!

Lara's anxieties concerning the interview situation have, based on previous experiences and perceived negative interactions, intensified over time. The enormity of anticipated interaction highlights how every action is perceived as symbolic of her "incompetence" and inability to perform "correctly" in social space, leaving her vulnerable to – certainly in her own estimation – to negative judgement and scrutiny by others:

Lara: By the time the interview came round I was in such a state. I was in the waiting room with all the other candidates and I wanted to burst into tears. I knew I'd failed already. It was so horrible I took a panic attack. My symptoms are visible too, physically trembling, sweating and I had a heavy tightness in my chest, blurry vision and so I felt like everyone could see me freaking out.

Louise: Then what happened?

Lara: I left. I felt like I didn't belong there. I couldn't sit in the interview in that state; I was a total wreck.

For Lara, the interview process becomes an emotionally charged, complex situation. The visceral experience of her sweaty, trembling and tense anxious bodies gives rise to a heightened sense of bodily self-awareness, a sensation then extending out into a reading of the space that the body occupies, thereby further amplifying the experience of distress that she reports about this attempt to access the workplace. This loss of bodily control and "inability" to self-regulate spiralling emotional experiences, particularly in the professional and formal setting of the interview/workplace, are deemed contextually "inappropriate".

Gwen works full-time in a job that provides her with routine and financial stability. Although her social anxieties do not completely restrict her ability to work, she recognises that they have had a detrimental impact on her occupational functioning and long-term career aspirations. Currently, she feels she is unable to progress further within her current role:

> Because of my SA I wouldn't cope with a job that required regular contact with other people e.g. working in a team or dealing with the public. Jobs that say 'must have an outgoing personality and be a team player!' They're not for me. This job allows me to avoid talking to people when I'm feeling particularly anxious.
>
> (Gwen, IR)

The workplace can be an intensely social environment and workplace culture may be further disabling. Wilson-Cortijo (2016, n.p.) argues that:

> In the past I imagine it would have been quite easy for a socially anxious individual to make a life for themselves doing some form of manual labour that wouldn't require the cultivation of 'people skills'. But in today's neoliberal world, where selling one's personal (communicative and performative) attributes are of the utmost importance, such skills are an absolute necessity. Whether it is in a corporate environment (meetings, group presentations, conferences, the importance of "leadership") or an ordinary retail job, there is a clear correlation between success and one's ability to produce confident spiel.

Gwen notes that the culture of her workplace, including expectations from colleagues to be sociable, is a significant factor in triggering her social anxieties:

> I find it difficult to socialise with colleagues [in the office]. I work on an open plan floor and I find this very stressful at times especially when it's busy and I feel more anxious. Comments have been made about how quiet I am and it has become an issue for me at times. There is an expectation for people to be outgoing and, although management are aware of my SA they don't always seem to understand situations that can affect my anxiety.
>
> (Gwen, IR)

Over time, Gwen has negotiated the workplace, employing certain strategies to manage her surroundings and by extension her social anxiety. Communal workspaces encourage what she refers to as "uncontrolled" social interactions and create an environment where she feels under "constant observation", so she deliberately blocks out her surrounding environment by wearing headphones, restricting external interferences and placing a barrier between her and any potential interactions, enabling her to focus on specific tasks and responsibilities:

> I've found coping mechanisms to deal with my anxiety but some days are better than others. I wear headphones all day to limit social contact with people and am able to focus on my work. I have my lunch on my own at a quiet time at the same time every day because, even though it's monotonous, it's familiar and makes me feel calmer [...]
>
> I sometimes go outside work for a walk at lunchtime during the summer months. I also go to the toilet and take a few minutes to do visualisation. If anything disrupts my routine e.g. a meeting [that] runs over my normal lunchtime, my anxiety increases greatly and I start to shake, my throat feels tight and I feel a need to escape.

Within her working environment, Gwen is able to manage her anxieties and limit her social interactions, but doing so is contingent upon numerous internal and external factors, including the fluctuating nature of her social anxiety and disruptions to her daily routine, matters that are not always within her control.

Kirsty is in full-time employment, and, in attempting to negotiate her social anxiety in the workplace, particular accommodations have been made that enable her to maintain employment. Unfortunately, though, those accommodations do sometimes cause tensions to arise with colleagues:

Kirsty: On a particularly bad day [at work] I might need to take a few 'time-outs' over and above my breaks to sort of compose myself and gather my thoughts, usually when I'm on the brink of freaking out and I'm getting flustered. I'll take a break. I try to put it off for as long as possible so people don't think I'm skiving[12] [...] They probably think I'm taking the piss[13] but sometimes I just need five minutes to reset, that's all.

Louise: Does that make it worse, that they might think that of you?

K: Without a doubt.

However, despite disclosing her social anxiety to her manager, who is "pretty understanding", enabling workplace accommodations to be made, Kirsty still feels that she is under surveillance by her colleagues, increasing the social intensity of her job. Her experience highlights that employers making adjustments within the workplace does not necessarily create an accommodating workplace culture among colleagues, which may be perceived as special treatment and delegitimised due to the relative invisibility of social anxiety (Richardson, 2005). Kirsty's work colleagues are indeed aware that specific accommodations have been made but are unsure of the exact circumstances under which they have been granted. Dunstan and Maceachen (2014) explore the issue of "external validity", through which certain accommodations may be resented, when there is a disjuncture between the visibility of the accommodations, such as regular "time outs", and the relative invisibility of the condition, as in the case of Kirsty's social anxiety.

Disclosure is a necessary step before requesting workplace accommodations, but the decision – itself highly anxiety-provoking – to disclose/conceal their "hidden" health condition may have a marked impact on their social relations or levels of functioning. Dyck and Jongbloed (2000), examining the workplace experiences of women with Multiple Sclerosis (MS), note that concealment of health conditions is easier if individuals are relatively free of supervision, crucial for the socially anxious precisely because the reality – or even just the possibility – of "over-sight", being surveyed and judged, is such a pernicious driver of their anxiety. For some, there is diminishing access to and status in the workplace in relation to disability (Imrie, 2001), chronic illness and returning to work after an injury (Crooks and Chouinard, 2006). Carol (QR) shifted from full-time employment to unemployment for a period of time and subsequently began re-gaining part-time employment:

> I was fired from a job [...] because of social anxiety and stress. Some co-workers tended not to respect my work abilities. Soon after that, I applied for and started to receive disability [benefits]. Now, I work just a few hours a week because interacting for several hours with the intensity of doing my job and being with others is just too difficult. I am more successful when I work fewer hours and have some ability to make decisions about how much to work.

Facey and Eakin (2010) discuss the contingent nature of work for people experiencing ill health. Contingent work here refers to part-time, casual, contract, temporary and self-employment forms of work that are often unstable and inconsistent, and yet may be the *only* forms of work – and workplace arrangement – with which people enduring social anxiety may be able to cope. Wilton (2004) notes similar issues for people with disabilities, where there may be "flexibility" within the workplace but often no "accommodation", but the root issue is much the same: namely, that workplaces remain hostile and unforgiving environments for people with many varieties of mental and physical difference, even if they may, under proper accommodations, still be able to "perform well" as workers. The challenges of social anxiety have rarely been considered in this connection, but participants in this study make abundantly clear that, even if they can control their anxiety sufficiently to make it into a workplace – and beyond the interview – there are still manifold socio-spatial micro-obstacles to their making a success of the experience.

Concluding remarks

This chapter has highlighted the spatial contingencies of social anxiety with respond to both home spaces and workplaces. By engaging with spaces of home and work it has demonstrated how uncertainty and ambivalence emerge and the multiple ways in which these spaces may be managed and/or renegotiated. The home is often considered a space to anchor, offering seemingly impenetrable protection from the outside world. The questionnaire responses met with these basic, potentially taken-for-granted assumptions of home as a safe space, but what emerged in subsequent conversations with participants is a more nuanced, ambivalent and often disruptive tale (Crooks, 2010). In the first instance, home operates as a space through which personal and material boundaries can be established, controlled and defended, but seemingly unremarkable and everyday objects are symbolic of the "outside" social world encroaching into one's personal and physical space, as well as a failure of the home to maintain these boundaries between inside and outside. "Home-making" often entails a continual practice of re-establishing bodily and home boundaries through routine and habitual practice: doing the "little things" as Karen (IR) tellingly puts it. Crucially, it is often a space-within-the-home, usually a bedroom, that offers the individual the strongest sense of safety and security, alluding to an ever-shrinking set of geographies within which the socially anxious person may feel at ease Chapter 7.

The workplace also becomes a key site of contention: on the one hand, it is recognised for its role in the process of recovery from ill health in providing routine and structure, as well as potentially promoting health and wellbeing; on the other, it is a place fraught with social interactions, performances and the potential for failure and embarrassment. Thus, consideration is often given by participants to the hiring process, mobility, workplace culture, the timing, spacing and pacing of the work environment (Hansen and Philo, 2007), and also colleague attitudes (particularly in relation to issues of disclosure). For many, even making it through the door of a workplace, even just to be interviewed, is hard enough, whereas for others maintaining employment – merely surviving let alone thriving – brings its own nagging demands and strains. It hardly needs underlining, but the difficult social geographies narrated in this chapter of home and work under the cloud of social anxiety disclose a substantial "impoverishment" of life quality for very many people today. This chapter has therefore laid the foundations for considering the next "layer" of this geography of social anxiety, but the next chapter seeks to delve deeper into these contingencies, embedding them within a wider network of interpersonal, social and spatial relations.

Notes

1 This chapter in the original thesis also focused on spaces of education but in the interests of space this section has been removed from the book.
2 Known in the sense it has been disclosed to employers and accommodations may have been implemented.

3 There have been parallels drawn between the routine, but restricted, daily geographies of people with social anxiety and those experienced globally by whole populations during the COVID-19 pandemic, specifically related to "social distancing", restrictions in mobility and social isolation.
4 Expressing negative emotion and dislike of the situation.
5 Sad face with two mouths for emphasis.
6 Community Psychiatric Nurse.
7 Bankey (1999) discusses these domestic and gendered relations in the context of agoraphobia, but the distinction between agoraphobia and social anxiety, as noted in Chapter 2, is "rather arbitrary". I might add that, while agreeing entirely with Bankey about the problematic gendered ideologies at play that arguably contribute to the likes of Karen's social anxiety, I cannot but also see strength – even dignity – in her efforts to reclaim a "good mother" role through the home-based resources and practices that *are* available to her (and hence to counter how her social anxiety makes her feel "less than").
8 The idea of anticipatory objects is normally mobilised in geography under wider considerations of anticipatory practices that create, predict and govern the "future" (Anderson, 2010), and includes attention to material objects (digital or physical), for example, nanotechnologies and other technoscientific assemblages for managing future threats (Anderson, 2007) such as climate change (Leyshon, Née and Geoghegan, 2012); and pre-emptive strategies and policy-making shaped by logics of risk and uncertainty (Evans, 2010).
9 Scots. "The close" is a communal stairwell or hallway in a block of flats and is sometimes used to refer to the whole block.
10 Electronic entry system/intercom for flats.
11 Agitated, excitable in a negative way.
12 Taking an undeserved break or avoidance of work duties.
13 Taking advantage of a situation for personal gain.

References

Anderson, B. (2007) 'Hope for nanotechnology: anticipatory knowledge and the governance of affect', *Area*, 39(3), pp. 156–165. https://doi.org/10.1111/j.1475-4762.2007.00743.x

Anderson, B. (2010) 'Preemption, precaution, preparedness: Anticipatory action and future geographies', *Progress in Human Geography*, 34(6), pp. 777–798. https://doi.org/10.1177/0309132510362600

Bankey, R. (1999) *The Paradox of Panic: A Geographic Analysis of Agoraphobic Experiences*. Ottawa: Carleton University.

Bennett, K. (2011) 'Homeless at home in East Durham', *Antipode*, 43(4), pp. 960–985. https://doi.org/10.1111/j.1467-8330.2010.00788.x

Beynon, P. and Tucker, S. (2006) Ill health, disability, benefit and work: A summary of recent research. *Social Policy Journal of New Zealand*, 29, pp. 78–101.

Bodden, S. et al. (2022) *Winter worries: understanding experiences of seasonal affective disorder in the UK through the 2022 'Big SAD Survey'*. Interim project report.

Bordo, S., Klein, B. and Silverman, M.K. (1998) 'Missing kitchens', in H.J. Nast and S. Pile (eds) *Places Through the Body*. London: Routledge, pp. 54–68.

Burch, L. (2023) '"I haven't got anywhere safe": disabled people's experiences of hate and violence within the home', *Social & Cultural Geography*, pp. 1–18. https://doi.org/10.1080/14649365.2023.2242325

Collier, E., Skitt, G. and Cutts, H. (2003) 'A study on the experience of insomnia in a psychiatric inpatient population', *Journal of Psychiatric and Mental Health Nursing*, 10(6), pp. 697–704. https://doi.org/10.1046/j.1365-2850.2003.00654.x

Crooks, V.A. (2010) 'Women's changing experiences of the home and life inside it after becoming chronically ill,' in Chouinard, V., Hall, E., and Wilton, R. (eds) *Towards Enabling Geographies: 'Disabled' Bodies and Minds in Society and Space*. London: Ashgate Publishing, pp. 45–62.

Crooks, V.A. and Chouinard, V. (2006) 'An embodied geography of disablement: Chronically ill women's struggles for enabling places in spaces of health care and daily life', *Health & Place*, 12(3), pp. 345–352. https://doi.org/10.1016/j.healthplace.2005.02.006

Davidson, J. (2000) '"… the world was getting smaller": Women, agoraphobia and bodily boundaries', *Area*, 32(1), pp. 31–40.

Davidson, J. (2009) 'Phobias and safekeeping: Emotions, selves and spaces', in S.J. Smith et al. (eds) *The SAGE Handbook of Social Geographies*. London: SAGE Publications Ltd, p. Chapter 16.

Davidson, J. and Henderson, V.L. (2010) '"Coming out" on the spectrum: autism, identity and disclosure', *Social & Cultural Geography*, 11(2), pp. 155–170. https://doi.org/10.1080/14649360903525240

Dunstan, D.A. and Maceachen, E. (2014) 'A theoretical model of co-worker responses to work reintegration processes', *Journal of Occupational Rehabilitation*, 24(2), pp. 189–198. https://doi.org/10.1007/s10926-013-9461-x

Dupuis, A. and Thorns, D.C. (1998) 'Home, home ownership and the search for ontological security', *The Sociological Review*, 46(1), pp. 24–47. https://doi.org/10.1111/1467-954X.00088

Dyck, I. (1998) 'Women with disabilities and everyday geographies: home space and the contested body', in R.A. Kearns and W.M. Gesler (eds) *Putting Health into Place: Landscape, Identity, and Well-being*. Syracuse, NY: Syracuse University Press, pp. 102–109.

Dyck, I. (1999) 'Body Troubles: Women, the Workplace and Negotiations of a Disabled Identity', in *Mind and Body Spaces*. London: Routledge.

Dyck, I. and Jongbloed, L. (2000) 'Women with multiple sclerosis and employment issues: a focus on social and institutional environments', *Canadian Journal of Occupational Therapy. Revue Canadienne D'ergotherapie*, 67(5), pp. 337–346. https://doi.org/10.1177/000841740006700506

Evans, B. (2010) 'Anticipating fatness: childhood, affect and the pre-emptive "war on obesity"', *Transactions of the Institute of British Geographers*, 35(1), pp. 21–38. https://doi.org/10.1111/j.1475-5661.2009.00363.x

Evans, J. and Wilton, R. (2016) '"I'm a better person when i'm working": Supportive workplaces, mental illness, and recover', in M.D. Giesbrecht and V. Crooks (eds) *Place, Health, and Diversity Learning from the Canadian Experience*. London: Routledge (Geographies of Health Series).

Evans, J. and Wilton, R. (2019) 'Well enough to work? Social enterprise employment and the geographies of Mental health recovery', *Annals of the American Association of Geographers*, 109(1), pp. 87–103. https://doi.org/10.1080/24694452.2018.1473753

Facey, M.E. and Eakin, J.M. (2010) 'Contingent work and ill-health: Conceptualizing the links', *Social Cognitive Theory*, 8, pp. 326–349. https://doi.org/10.1057/sth.2010.3

Grove, B., Secker, J. and Seebohm, P. (2005) *New Thinking about Mental Health and Employment*. Radcliffe Publishing.

Hansen, N. and Philo, C. (2007) 'The normality of doing things differently: Bodies, spaces and disability geography', *Tijdschrift voor Economische en Sociale Geografie*, 98(4), pp. 493–506. https://doi.org/10.1111/j.1467-9663.2007.00417.x

Himle, J.A. et al. (2014) 'A comparison of unemployed job-seekers with and without social anxiety', *Psychiatric services (Washington, D.C.)*, 65(7), pp. 924–930. https://doi.org/10.1176/appi.ps.201300201

Imrie, R. (2001). 'Barriered and bounded places and the spatialities of disability', *Urban Studies*, 38, 231–237. https://doi.org/10.1080/00420980124639

Ingold, T. (2007) 'Materials against materiality', *Archaeological Dialogues*, 14(1), pp. 1–16. https://doi.org/10.1017/S1380203807002127

Kane, M. (2023) 'The violent uncanny: Exploring the material politics of austerity', *Political Geography*, 102, p. 102843. https://doi.org/10.1016/j.polgeo.2023.102843

Larsen, I.B., Bøe, T.D. and Topor, A. (2020) 'Things matter: about materiality and recovery from mental health difficulties', *International Journal of Qualitative Studies on Health and Well-being*, 15(1). https://doi.org/10.1080/17482631.2020.1802909

Laws, J. (2013). 'Recovery work' and 'magic' among long-term mental health service-users', *The Sociological Review*, 61, pp. 344–362. https://doi.org/10.1111/1467-954X.12020

Leyshon, C., Née, B. and Geoghegan, H. (2012) 'Anticipatory objects and uncertain imminence: cattle grids, landscape and the presencing of climate change on the Lizard Peninsula, UK', *Area*, 44(2), pp. 237–244.

Martin, E.N. (2021) *Mental ill-health and experiences of work in a.* Unpublished PhD Thesis. University of Glasgow.

Masters, K. (2021) *Putting the 'Social' in 'Social Anxiety Disorder': Exploring Women's Experiences from a Feminist and Anti-Psychiatry Perspective.* Unpublished PhD Thesis. University of Birmingham.

McKee, K., Soaita, A.M. and Hoolachan, J. (2020) '"Generation rent" and the emotions of private renting: self-worth, status and insecurity amongst low-income renters', *Housing Studies*, 35(8), pp. 1468–1487. https://doi.org/10.1080/02673037.2019.1676400

Mclean, D.J. (2008a) 'Authors meet critics: reviews and response, review 3', *Social & Cultural Geography*, 9(5), pp. 557–572. https://doi.org/10.1080/14649360802224721

Mclean, D.J. (2008b) 'Reviews in brief: Home. By Alison Blunt and Robyn Dowling. Review no. 3, London/New York: Routledge. 2006', *Cultural Geographies*, 15(3), pp. 397–397. https://doi.org/10.1177/14744740080150030703

Miller, D. (Ed.), (2001) *Home Possessions: Material Culture behind Closed Doors.* Oxford: Berg Publishers.

Moore, J. (2000) 'Placing home in context', *Journal of Environmental Psychology*, 20(3), pp. 207–217. https://doi.org/10.1006/jevp.2000.0178

Moss, P. (1997) 'Negotiating spaces in home environments: Older women living with arthritis', *Social Science & Medicine*, 45(1), pp. 23–33. https://doi.org/10.1016/S0277-9536(96)00305-X

Parr, H., Philo, C. and Burns, N. (2003) '"That awful place was home": Reflections on the contested meanings of Craig Dunain Asylum', *Scottish Geographical Journal*, 119(4), pp. 341–360. https://doi.org/10.1080/00369220318737183

Philo, C., Parr, H. and Burns, N. (2005) '"An oasis for us": "in-between" spaces of train-ing for people with mental health problems in the Scottish Highlands', *Geoforum*, 36(6), pp. 778–791. https://doi.org/10.1016/j.geoforum.2005.01.002

Porteous, J.D. (1976) 'Home: The territorial core', *Geographical Review*, 66(4), pp. 383–390. https://doi.org/10.2307/213649

Richardson, J.C. (2005) 'Establishing the (extra)ordinary in chronic widespread pain', *Health (London, England: 1997)*, 9(1), pp. 31–48. https://doi.org/10.1177/1363459305048096

Schmied, V. and Kearney, E. (2018) *Reconceptualising Mothering Narratives*. Penrith: University of Western Sydney.

Segrott, J. and Doel, M.A. (2004) 'Disturbing geography: obsessive-compulsive disor-der as spatial practice', *Social & Cultural Geography*, 5(4), pp. 597–614. https://doi.org/10.1080/1464936042000317721

Smith, N.D. (2013) *The everyday social geographies of living with epilepsy*. PhD. University of Glasgow. https://eleanor.lib.gla.ac.uk/record=b3004343 (Accessed: 26 May 2023).

Stravynski, A. (2014) *Social Phobia: An Interpersonal Approach*. Cambridge: Cambridge University Press.

Valentine, G. (1998) '"Sticks and stones may break my bones": A personal geography of harassment', *Antipode*, 30(4), pp. 305–332. https://doi.org/10.1111/1467-8330.00082

Warrington, M. (2001) '"I must get out": The geographies of domestic violence', *Transactions of the Institute of British Geographers*, 26(3), pp. 365–382. https://doi.org/10.1111/1475-5661.00028

Wilson-Cortijo, S. (2016) 'Social anxiety ruined my life – until I found the one place I felt at home', *The Guardian Online*, https://www.theguardian.com/comment isfree/2016/jan/19/social-anxiety-disorder-suicidal-city#comments, Accessed 10 Feb-ruary 2021.

Wilton, R. (2004) 'From flexibility to accommodation? Disabled people and the rein-vention of paid work', *Transactions of the Institute of British Geographers*, 29, pp. 420–432. https://doi.org/10.1111/j.0020-2754.2004.00139.x

7   Spatialities of social anxiety II

Diminishing social worlds

Social anxiety has made my world so much smaller.

(Anna, QR)

Introduction

The aim of this chapter is to deepen the accounts from Spatialities I (Chapter 6) focusing on the relational and embodied encounters and reactions, and the micro-textures of these encounters that comprise anxious experiences. Participants' social worlds uncover the complexity in, and limitations placed on, everyday social life. They also highlight the broader impact over a life course as opportunities for encounter, both passing and sustained, become increasingly diminished. Significantly, participants expressed difficulty with numerous aspects of social life and relationships, inclusive of the close social interactions, bonds and support with family and friends as well as the wider interactions and encounters that comprise everyday life and spaces. Despite the importance of social encounters to psychosocial wellbeing and quality of life, few studies have examined how social anxieties shape social worlds. Then, this chapter turns to the anxieties associated with public spaces and (im)mobilities associated with public transport. Of key consideration is how individual's social geographies are disabled or become diminished to "predictable, purposeful trips, origins and destinations" in the face of mobilities experienced as "a messy, unpredictable, diverse and changeable reality" (Huxley 1997 p. 2 *cited in* Imrie, 2000, p. 1641).

Friendships and family relations

Friendships and family relations are significant social relationships that form the structure of our daily lives (Pahl, 2000). The strong interpersonal bonds integral to these relations are crucial for managing and maintaining physical and mental health by providing fundamental sources of emotional, instrumental and informational support (Tough, Siegrist and Fekete, 2017). Many respondents note a substantial decline in the quality of interpersonal relations

DOI: 10.4324/9781003206880-7

with both family and friends. Participants note that the disintegration of social relations occurs "over time", "gradually" and "to the point where I faded away [from social life]" (Grace QR, Claire, QR; Kirsty, QR). Four interrelated themes were identified that capture the processes involved in participants' diminishing or changing social relationships: difficulty and uncertainty, opportunities available for social contact and the emotional work involved in sustaining relationships.

Difficulty and uncertainty

The progression of social anxiety is associated with increased socio-spatial isolation as patterns of social interaction change and use of public space are encountered with great difficulty or avoided completely (Dyck, 1995). Smart et al. (2012, p. 99) explore some of the difficult dimensions of negotiating friendships, arguing that while they may provide a sense of ontological security through mutually supportive and beneficial interactions and a strengthening of self and collective identity, they can also be "ontologically unsettling":

> Relationships with family and friends have taken a big hit over the last few years. I've slowly withdrawn as social things became increasingly difficult. I have no friends, I slowly pushed them away [by] rearranging [plans] and not turning up – I didn't want to burden them with my problems. I was constantly making excuses. The longer I didn't see them the more anxious I was. I was afraid of losing them. I felt incredibly guilty and undeserving, I wasn't being a good or a true friend, that I was avoiding them, but I was even more afraid of being judged by them and of going outside and being surrounded by people I didn't know.
>
> (Leanne, QR)

Social relations are deeply entangled with the "self", thus, the physical and emotional need to distance oneself from the objects of anxiety that completely undermine any sense of self is complex. Leanne's (QR) gradual disengagement from social life is implemented as a self-protective strategy (Chapter 8). Crucially, this is also entangled with her "moral worth and ethical standing" (Smart et al., 2012, p. 107), one in which she believes she is "undeserving" of her friendships. Smart et al. (2012) view friendship as the mirror through which we face ourselves but, for those highly sensitive to such interpersonal dynamics, the difficulties inherent in social relations are that they provide a painfully close channel for unearthing the precariousness of the self.

Fewer opportunities

Due to the difficulties and uncertainties faced by participants in their relationships with family and friends, there are fewer opportunities for social contact.

This decrease in social contact contributes greatly to participant's experiences of loneliness and isolation:

> As my social anxiety got worse, I started to get more insular. The more intense it got over a longer period of time I started to feel very lonely and isolated. Before, I would avoid going to the shops or getting the bus during rush hour because there were too many people but the longer it went on the more it started to affect work and close relationships and friendships [...] so my social life has, well, I don't really have one.
>
> (Anna, QR)

Similarly, Gillian is frustrated that she is missing opportunities for bonding and social activities with close friends and, as a result, feels isolated. However, she also recognises the locations and frequency of social contact are unmanageable for her:

> I'm fortunate enough to have a few close friends who I now see occasionally but I often feel left out. They are a much closer group and have been on holiday and go out regularly together, go for lunch and things like that, all things I feel I've really missed out on. Even though I'd love to go out with them I can't bring myself to meet up with them 2-3 times a week like they do. It's far too much for me. It's really overwhelming to be in a bar or a cafe, there's so many things involved and too much to consider going to places like that or just going out, really.
>
> (Gillian, QR)

Gillian's experience is emblematic of the gradual restrictions placed on sociospatial life as certain interactions and spaces become out of bounds. Her experience of missing out leaves her feeling excluded and detached from the main group, creating, in turn, fewer opportunities for social interaction.

Emotional work

Simply interacting with other people can have a negative impact on some participants' overall sense of wellbeing. Participants describe the emotional cost of social interaction as "debilitating" (Simon, QR), "overwhelming" (Dawn, QR) and "exhausting and a constant battle" (Dawn, QR). Several respondents commented that not only was there a societal stigma surrounding mental health, but people close to them were frequently questioning why they could not "snap out of it" for the sake of children or their job. A person's struggle to "get well" (Karen, IR) led to further questions about how much someone wants to get well, particularly when they engage in destructive behaviours, miss or avoid doctor's appointments or relapse. While crucial sources of emotional aid, developing new and maintaining existing social relationships requires considerable amounts of emotional work (Bilecen, 2014). Marta (QR) explains:

> I'm constantly on edge whenever I leave my home. [...] Every time I interact with someone. I'm constantly conscious of how I look, where my hands are, whether I'm making enough/too much eye contact, what they're thinking of me, if my voice is shaking, if they can tell I'm nervous, if I'm going to make a fool of myself and how I'm supposed to pluck up the courage to ask or say what I need to [say]. It is completely and utterly draining.

These transient and seemingly insignificant micro-interactions result in a state akin to an interpersonal "burnout". Burnout, most associated with occupational stress, is characterised by emotional, mental or physical exhaustion that "originates from emotionally demanding interpersonal relationships" with others (Maslach, 1993, p. 18):

> Since [school], I've had no friends at all. I've never attempted to make any, because I simply don't know how to, and even if I did, I don't know what it's like to have a friend, like how to behave. I feel the pressures of having a friend [would be that] I would have to go out regularly and interact with [them]. It is not worth the effort.
>
> (Marta, QR)

Marta highlights her deep-set belief that she is incapable of making friends and lacks the necessary social skills to interact with other people. Equally, she attributes the absence of interpersonal relationships with negative aspects of the self. She expresses a deep sense of shame and perceives the lack of close social bonds to be a personal failure:

> I thought my inability to function properly in social situations was just because I was broken somehow or plain pathetic and I had no friends or social life because I was a horrible person (Marta QR).

When asked to consider how her social anxiety affects her day-to-day life, Priya states she spends most of her time "avoiding people, even friends, [and] alienating myself as I feel such toxic shame" (Priya, QR). The paralysing capacity of shame is entrenched in an inherent sense of self-worthlessness.

Loneliness and social isolation

The pervasive nature of loneliness and social isolation is evident through the questionnaire and interview responses. In the questionnaires, there are 21 references to being alone, feeling lonely and loneliness and 46 references to feeling isolated, isolating and isolation. While research alludes to how social exclusion and isolation can embed loneliness, the situated and embodied experience of loneliness remains something of an academic "blind spot" in human geography. The social dimensions of loneliness and isolation are associated with a lack of meaningful social connections and wider networks of support. Weiss (1973) developed two distinct forms of loneliness: emotional loneliness and social loneliness. The former describes the lack or loss of intimate social relations with family, friends or a partner. The latter is associated with the absence of a wider social network or system of support. The following addresses a relational perspective, taking into consideration the interplay of emotional and social forces that create and sustain experiences of loneliness. Dawn expands on her feelings of loneliness:

> I am extremely lonely all of the time. Being too afraid to leave the house resulted in me losing all of my friends at one point in time as [I] often face problems when going out and trying to get in contact [with them] I become extremely agitated and nervous. This can lead to me avoiding contact altogether for long periods of time and becoming even more isolated.
>
> (Dawn, QR)

Structural barriers can also embed and exacerbate loneliness (Olfson et al., 2000) including stigmatising attitudes to mental health and low professional and public recognition (NICE, 2013) (Chapter 5). Simon (QR) recounts his experience of social isolation and loneliness in relation to healthcare systems and wider society:

> From my earliest days at school, I was seen as 'different' and isolated. Despite the school's insistence that I see a number of child psychologists, none were able to offer anything by way of help [...] I was denied access to the NHS completely [and] I remained isolated for most of my life. [...] I moved [away from home], where I became even more isolated than in the past. I joined a [support] group. It took many years to change my experience with social anxiety [...] but at times it seems that I hadn't made enough changes to be accepted and despite everyone knowing why I was 'weird', I was told that I wasn't welcome at the [social anxiety] meetups. I thought about taking my life several times, I felt alone, isolated, hopeless—I saw no point in my existence.

Simon's painful emotional and social loneliness is compounded by structural barriers that exclude him further from social and civic life including significant failures by healthcare professionals to provide information or a diagnosis, a stringent lack of mental health support services and stigmatising attitudes within the community. Frie (2017, p. 26) suggests experiences of "loneliness may reflect the emotional dynamic of a person's inner life or be a response to the loss of relatedness and a hostile social environment". Despite finding local user-led support groups,

Simon was too "weird" and too "different" to participate, straddling a contested boundary between "normal" behaviour and social "deviance" (Busfield, 2017). This experience echoes Parr's (2000, p. 235) assessment of mental health drop-in centres, in which more or less acceptable ways of being are "constructed and maintained" through the licensing of "certain behaviours and emotions".

Third places

Throughout the questionnaires and interviews, participants reflect on their feelings of safety in specified sites and settings across public space particularly those that support daily routines and wider social and civic life. Participants also expand on their experiences with specific reference to other sites of social-ising and enjoyment including, but not limited to, cinemas, theatres, cafes, lunch halls, libraries, gyms, social groups and museums. Informal gatherings and shared spaces, which Jeffres et al. (2009, p. 334) refer to as "third places", operate as "unique public spaces of social interaction providing context for sociability, spontaneity, community building and emotional expressiveness" beyond the home (the first place) and work (the second place) (Oldenburg, 1999) (Chapter 6). This research has also focused on the significance of third places in promoting and maintaining health and wellbeing (Butterfield and Martin, 2016) as spaces that help to foster interpersonal relationships and pro-mote a sense of self, community and connection. The therapeutic qualities of third places facilitate health, healing and restoration as places that "remedy or prevent emotional loneliness, not just through companionship, but more importantly through personal and emotional support" (Glover and Parry, 2009, p. 104). Furthermore, these places, situated on peoples' everyday maps, offer a temporary escape from the stressors of everyday life that can provide a sense of emotional relief and regulation. Overwhelmingly, participants express difficulty in developing and maintaining social bonds and interpersonal rela-tionships with friends and family. The following reflects not only the magni-tude of social and public spaces that people with social anxiety deem "out of bounds", but the specificities of individual experience that render certain inter-actions and performances associated with these spaces as inherently distress-ing. Practices of shopping, purchasing items, engaging with supermarket workers and shopping centre/supermarket spaces all presented as considerable sources of anxiety for participants. Feminist geographers have paid consider-able attention to the associations between women's fear and experiences of panic in the context of consumer spaces to uncover how spaces with no dis-cernible danger present a considerable loss of control to bodily and spatial boundaries (Davidson, 2000).

Consumer spaces

Davidson (2001) argues that consumer spaces present "grave dangers" for ago-raphobic women as they enter a "feminised" space, one which constructs "feminised" identities, or more accurately "ideals", that they are expected to assume through consumption. Yet, like accounts of social anxiety, women became intimately aware of "our-selves", critically so. Consumer spaces, whether shopping malls or supermarkets, are inherently contradictory as "marketing strategies often make extensive use of ideas about gender, simultaneously addressing women as consumers and objectifying women's bodies" (Bondi and Davidson, 2008). Hickinbottom-Brawn (2013, p. 737) suggests that consumer culture and the psy-disciplines have enabled social phobias and anxieties to flourish by "shap[ing] self-understandings and promot[ing] regulative ideals for living." They uncover a much wider sociocultural progression of social anxiety in the era of "neoliberal enterprise culture" where personal value is shaped and defined by patterns of consumption. Arguing that "shame-based advertising, aimed to heighten awareness of offensive aspects of self" (2013, p. 727), guides consumers towards consumption that leaves no room for unhappiness or psychological and emotional distress. In a similar vein, Jackson and Everts (2010) approach social anxiety as a "social condition" as opposed to an individual experience, exploring how everyday practices of consumption are disrupted in the context of food- related anxieties. Crucially, they highlight how anxiety manifests through practice, in decisions to consume (or not consume), for example, particular food products. The central concern raised by Jackson and Everts is that "some of the very practices that constitute our everyday lives [are the ones] whose disruption further entrenches those anxieties" (2010, p. 2802).

Bondi and Davidson (2008, p. 22) report similar experiences by women living with agoraphobia where intensely gendered consumer spaces, conveying messages of self-improvement, "stir up troubling emotions and associations for many women". This gendering of space is also evident in experiences of social anxiety as consumer spaces, including supermarkets, shopping centres and retail stores, which are strongly associated with negative judgements, and episodes of panic and are spaces in which respondents are "overwhelmed by choice, [a feeling of] not being able to escape" (Anna, QR) and a "pressure to buy things" (Sarah, QR). Supermarkets can be extremely overwhelming and disorientating, with Davidson (2000, p. 31) highlighting the "disturbing architecture" of mall spaces. She states that "[t]hey are assemblages of numerous and overlaid attempts at sensory stimulation which can render the atmosphere excruciatingly intense":

[My] anxiety peaks in the supermarket (or at the thought of going to the shops). It takes weeks for me to build up the courage to go and I'm forced when I'm basically running out of food. High ceilings and horrible lighting, I feel claustrophobic and get a kind of tunnel vision all at the same time, it's so disorientating.

(Claire, QR)

I cannot stand being in the supermarket, I cannot stand people being near me and find it really hard to cope when it's busy. I'll never shop at the weekends and will sometimes go out to do a shop at 11 or 12 at night to avoid the crowds.

(Kerrie, QR)

While neither male nor female respondents report feeling "very safe" in shopping centres, as a percentage of total respondents only 2.4% of female respondents report feeling "safe" compared to 20.5% of male respondents. Equally, participants who discussed anxieties in consumer spaces in the online questionnaire and interviews were predominantly female.

Karen's experience is particularly salient in demonstrating how her perceptions of, and relationship with, shopping and consumer spaces have changed as her social anxiety progressed:

Before this [anxiety] I was just a 'normal' person who did my own shopping every week, took my kids out, paid my own bills, I socialised – I was really sociable – with friends, we'd go to town once a month, shop, have lunch. Now, the thought of doing any of those things terrifies me ... having a panic attack in the middle of the shopping centre with people staring at me when I'm freaking out and screaming get me out of here! If [the children] need anything – pants, socks, new trainers – their Nanny[1] takes them 'cause I can't do any of that anymore.

(Karen, IR)

Habits and routines embedded in everyday life help to foster and sustain social relations with family and friends as well as shaping identity. Davidson (2001, p. 36) notes the difficulty faced by women with agoraphobia entering these "feminised sphere[s]" of life highlighting they "can neither 'do' the shopping (for necessities) or 'go' shopping (for pleasure or contact with friends)". Karen's routines of shopping and her perceptions of herself as "normal" and "sociable" are mutually reinforcing. Later in the interview, she expresses a deep sense of failure about not being able to provide adequately for her children and her dependence on her mother, who is now her carer (Chapter 6). She reflects fondly on "the old me" and although she "cannot understand how I got to this point", her anxieties have had a life-altering effect. The panic that Karen experiences in the shopping centre now is far removed from the enjoyable, sociable or even mundane associations that existed prior to the onset of her social anxiety. The annihilation of this once active sphere of life demonstrates not only how anxiety "disrupts the flow" of social and spatial life (Jackson and Everts, 2010, p. 2802) but has a significant impact on how she views herself as a parent, friend and daughter.

Winnicott (1971) argues that experience is shaped in "potential space", akin to a "third space", where the inner psychical and emotional realities of the individual and their external worlds intertwine. Zimmerman (1999), drawing on Winnicottian psychoanalysis, views public and civic space as a "potential space". Highly organised and privatised consumer spaces, carefully curated as public spaces, provide a platform for entertainment and socialising that enable the individual to "grow in value and self-regard" allowing "the (false) self to blossom as consumer" (Zimmerman, 1999, p. 570). Echoing Hickinbottom-Brawn (2013), consumer culture is largely concerned with the building or expanding of identities enabling the creation and presentation of a new and improved "self" to the world. Yet, for both Emma (QR) and Priya (QR), these spaces, where self and social identities must blend seamlessly with socially accepted norms and expectations, embody a sense of uncertainty, insecurity and anticipation:

> Supermarkets, shops [and] shopping centres, more than any other place[s], bring out the worst of my anxiety. I get embarrassed about what I buy and anxious that I'll be judged for my food choices. I won't buy something if I think it makes me look unhealthy or greedy. [It is] all made worse by waiting in line to pay and [the] attempts at small talk by the person at the checkout […]
>
> (Emma, QR)

> I will not go to places where there will be lots of people—e.g. I avoid going into a shop I previously wanted to go in if I see there is a long queue, or it is busy. I rarely buy things I want in front of friends or parents and have to arrange either to get them alone or order them off the internet, so I don't have to experience the fear of them watching me and possibly negatively judging me. I won't wear new clothes or t-shirts with words on them for fear of embarrassment.
>
> (Priya, QR)

What is clear is that respondents perceive consumer spaces to have the potential for negative interactions and attention. Indeed, these encounters make individuals feel noticed and "marked" fuelling feelings of self-consciousness and fear of judgement from other people. This is evident in anxieties that others will view Emma as "unhealthy" or "greedy" through her shopping habits and Priya's fear that her personal choices will invite possible scrutiny from strangers as well as family and/or friends. Southgate (2016, p. 246) argues that the ability to negotiate potential space "requires the capacity to tolerate its inherent ambiguity". Yet, it is precisely at this meeting point, between our inner and outer worlds, where anxieties emanate from, a place where social expectations, interactions and daily processes collide with an intense self-awareness and debilitating self-consciousness.

Public transport

By exploring anxious "(im)mobilities" through participants experiences on and perceptions of public transport, I do not intend to reinforce a binary that equates mobility with activity and immobility with passivity (Adey, 2017). Instead, by focussing on the relational contingencies between mobility and immobility, I aim to demonstrate how travelling between destinations is often fraught with difficulty and tension for those who experience social space as extremely invasive and complex. To contextualise this complexity, it is crucial to recognise the personal difficulties that people face in negotiating transit spaces in their everyday routines by unpacking the affective, embodied and relational dimensions of "journeying", while also highlighting the steps taken to mitigate anxieties and routine disruption. There are multiple factors that shape and influence the journey, including crowded conditions, unfamiliar routes, transfer requirements, fellow passengers and affective atmospheres, as well as the embodied aspects of people's social anxieties. Therefore, it is important to consider how the everyday experiences of travelling by public transport with proximate others unfold and the wider implications for an individual's daily and longer-term social geographies.

Travelling on public transport is highlighted in the online questionnaire as a situation provoking intense social anxieties for participants. Bissell (2010, p. 277) notes "that [the] experience of being with others in spaces of public transport" is particularly "uncongenial", as passengers are gripped by a sense of "unease" and "foreboding". Indeed, in an increasingly urbanised and busy world, the daily commute is rarely enjoyable for most people, as everyday frustrations, irritations and anxieties erupt. While these spaces are felt by some respondents to be so unsafe that they "avoid public transport almost completely" (Anna, QR), for others it is an unavoidable yet deeply disruptive component of everyday life. The spatial confines of transport spaces arguably mark a near-unique space in the public realm, one where people are often confined in an enclosed space in close proximity to unknown others for considerable periods of time. As Kim (QR) explains, "I feel very claustrophobic and panicky being in a small space with a lot of people, so the idea of being stuck on a crowded bus or train gives me the absolute fear." While being "stuck" is a temporary state between stops, locating spaces of safety is inherently difficult while "in transit", resulting in an urgent need to escape which, for practical and safety reasons, is impossible. Cara (QR) writes, "there's times where I've asked the driver to stop the bus to let me off [between stops] but they can't, so I just try to get a grip of myself and calm down." Others, recognising this temporary confinement, state, "once I'm on, I know I need to ride it out … so to speak" (Ben, IR). Mia (QR) provides an account of the internal conflicts and external tensions that arise while travelling by public transport, demonstrating how space and its associated mobilities, often perceived as "banal" (Binnie *et al.*, 2007) quickly become intolerable and distressing:

I hate having to buy a ticket [...] counting out the fare and my brain scrambles because there's a huge queue behind me and the bus driver is waiting [and] everyone is watching as I get on. Then, if someone [is] sitting next to me or it's packed, it gets too hot, I feel trapped to the point

I can't even say "excuse me" to get off and then [I] miss my stop. I have a bad reaction to small, closed in, packed spaces. I start to sweat [and] panic and then I feel sick, and I don't travel well anyway, so I'd usually start feeling really sick [...] Not knowing where to get off, having to stand up while the bus is moving, what if I fall? Am I going to panic with all these people are watching me? It's not even worth the hassle.

Beyond a "mere transition zone" (Hulme and Truch, 2006, p. 47) between origin and destination, the bus journey is a loaded time-space environment. There are a series of overlapping social, spatial and affective dimensions that result in Mia's reluctance to travel by bus, starting with the face-to-face interaction and social performance involved in the strikingly ordinary task of purchasing a ticket. There is an implicit pressure to board quickly and efficiently and failure to do so may draw the negative attention, even ire, of others. Bissell (2007, p. 285) argues that "there is a tendency to be quite unaware of one's body" while journeying "where the body remains passive and acquiescent" but said "passivity" is arguably far removed from Mia's experience of journeying, which not only mobilises very particular anxieties about being in close proximity to other people but also entails distressing corporeal awareness of the resulting bodily manifestations of those anxieties. Furthermore, the very conditions of travel indicate the ways in which bodies are open and responsive to our immediate socio-spatial surrounding. Take the shrinking of available space: this particularly salient component produces an atmospheric shift that "registers in and through sensing bodies while also remaining diffuse" (McCormack, 2008, p. 413). This shrinking, coupled with a felt increase in temperature, presses upon the body, giving rise to bodily sensations of sweat or panic through which a heightened sense of bodily awareness and the self-in-space emerges. In addition, fleeting interactions, in the form of a mumbled "excuse me", are rife with anxieties that are further exacerbated by the anticipation of "embarrassing" events – a stumble, a flush of panic – that will mark her presence in public space even more visible. Mia finds herself incapacitated by anxieties that register viscerally, rendering her body and its meeting with the surrounding environment completely outwith her control. She subsequently states that she will often "walk for 40 minutes instead of taking a 10-minute bus ride", highlighting the exhausting and time-consuming measures that are put into practice in order to mitigate the effects of such anxieties (Chapter 8).

Transport spaces become a contained microcosm of wider public space, serving to heighten already existing anxieties. People feel "out of place" and attuned to their anticipated and perceived transgressions from socially and culturally constructed "norms". Social codes and rituals serve to increase people's anxieties about "disturbing" others, anxieties that are somewhat magnified in enclosed spaces. Callum (IR), who marked public transport as "very unsafe" in the online questionnaire, refers to the public transport "code of conduct" and how this further complicates journeys:

> In general, it's just a painful experience. There's so many rules about what you should or shouldn't do; the "code of conduct" of the bus or whatever. I constantly think about whether I'm invading someone's personal space like, if there's no spare seats and [I] need to sit next to someone, I'm on the edge of my seat so I'm not touching them or too close [to them]. Also, I don't want the person sitting next to me feeling offended by [me] (probably blatantly) distancing myself from them.

Maintaining a relative distance from the people around him is important for Callum to ensure that he is not encroaching into other people's personal space (as opposed to other people violating his personal space). Goffman ascribes the term "civil inattention" to the socially constructed rituals of social space that encapsulate how individuals maintain a veneer of privacy by actively disengaging from one another. This ritual addresses the transient and fleeting nature of encounters with others as people acknowledge each other's presence through a glance or a faint smile, but then retreat. While Goffman's focus in these types of encounters is specular, Callum's concern is also one of proximity and whether he is seen to create too much distance between him and his co-commuters at the risk of appearing rude or causing offence. This distance, what Goffman terms "aversion", is a violation of civil inattention, where the individual is undeserving of even the most minimal acknowledgement. Arguably, Callum and others avoid such minimal acknowledgements as an act of self-preservation in the face of a debilitating sense of self-consciousness, rather than as an outright rejection of the other person. Goffman conceives the regulation of social encounters as a routine social norm ingrained into the practice of everyday life, but Giddens (1991, p. 123) argues that the practice "demands a chronic attention to detail" – an understanding that resonates more clearly with the experiences of people with social anxiety. In fact, the experience of commuting for most participants is only habitual in the sense that it occurs regularly and most experience journeys with great trepidation and unease. As a result, people engage in significant amounts of planning, and Mia (IR) explains the mindset of being able to "ride out" her journeys (mentioned above) by referring to the laborious planning engaged in beforehand:

> It takes a lot for me to get on in the first place, hours of planning and thinking things through, running through all the scenarios in my head, checking the route, how many stops before I get off and just knowing that it's going to be a really uncomfortable and stressful thing. It's a pure nightmare, I find the whole thing really overwhelming and stressful, but I got myself there.

Nina (IR) did not use public transport at all and would take the more expensive option of travelling by taxi. Now she uses the bus, however, like Mia, she goes to great lengths to limit any uncertainty associated with her journey:

> [I]f I have to travel, because my job involves having to visit people, I plan the routes really, really carefully and make sure I've got access to maps and Google and I know where the bus goes from and where it stops and all that, and how long it's going to take me to get there [...]. If, which happens quite frequently, if public transports doesn't turn up or is late [after] the extent I go to plan as rigorously as I do [...] It happened the other week; it's just a nightmare.

Spaces of public transport are frequently described as non-social environments, although they, like other public spaces of encounter, are primed for "potentially integrative events" (Laurier and Philo, 2006, p. 199). Conversational interactions appear to be uncommon, as participants rarely mentioned explicit instances where they encountered a problematic conversation with other passengers. With the exception of necessary social interactions with a driver or the pleasantries involved in negotiating crowded spaces, which are by no means insignificant (as is evident in Mia's narrative above), the interactions on public transport are relatively "uneventful".

As Bissell (2010, p. 271) notes that a tension "exists between the isolation of travelling unaccompanied [...] within a collective of other passengers". This collective dwelling disrupts expectations of rights to privacy in public and the "proxemic" rules that dictate how people perceive and organise their social and personal space. In an act of self-preservation, passengers attempt to extend the boundaries of personal space, creating what Goffman (1971) terms "territories of the self". Where creating physical distance is difficult, individuals seek socially and emotionally to disconnect from people around them:

> I use Google Maps and sort of follow my journey 'live', so I tune out and concentrate on my phone. It helps with a fear of getting lost or being stranded somewhere [...] I always wear headphones, people aren't likely to start any small talk with [me when I've got] headphones on and [I'm] zoned out, minding my own business type of thing. [The headphones] help to block everything out so I can just focus on my phone. (Craig, QR)

Passengers habitually fatigued and frustrated by the daily commute strive to be socially inaccessible, actively choosing seats in an empty row and using mobile technologies to disconnect from their surrounding environments. When there is such a pervasive feeling of uncertainty about journeying as described by Craig (and Nina, above), the use of "real-time" technology such as Google Maps enables him to monitor the progress of the journey and to pinpoint his exact location on the map, particularly in unfamiliar territory. Sound (and the "awkward silences") on public transport is implicit here in producing a heightened awareness that permeates individual experience, and so many participants often use headphones to dull the sensory experience of public space, creating a protective boundary as well as "marking" the body as "out of bounds" for interaction (but not necessarily "out of place"). These strategies are discussed further in Chapter 8.

Although planning is an exhausting and time-consuming practice, part of this preparation is about being able to mitigate the effects of unexpected interactions and events. Equally, people remain responsive to their surrounding environments and make last-minute changes in order "to sit on a quiet bus, rather than change tubes and battle through busy stations" or when the conditions for travel "just don't feel right" (Dina, QR). When considerable amounts of time are spent preparing for (even the most habitual of) journeys, there is spontaneity in being able to re-direct its course in response to often uncertain and changing conditions of travel. That said, the consequences of altering daily routines mean that it takes significantly longer to complete everyday tasks. Beth often wakes up "two hours early so my dad can take me to college on his way to work". Similarly, Greg (QR) writes, I can only get the bus to uni and it's really problematic. I tend to avoid rush hour but if I finish uni later, the buses are always packed. I usually wait a few hours and travel home later or get the night bus that's quieter. Dyck (1995, p. 310) notes that the use of "transportation, particularly in crowded, rush-hour conditions", is problematic for women living with chronic illness as they negotiate the social and physical environment between home and work. Lisa experiences similar disruptions in her day:

> I take the bus to university mostly every day and I hate it. I find myself jumping off and taking the next bus if it gets too busy or claustrophobic, but that usually makes me late for class and that makes me panic too. I can't win!

While seemingly ingrained into the habitual rhythm of social life, pervasive anxieties constitute and unsettle spaces of mobility, disrupting the experience of the daily commute as "the routine and repetitive transition from place to place: a transition ideally meant to be safe" (Bissell, Vannini and Jensen, 2017, p. 806). Consequently, people spend substantial amounts of energy simply getting to and from significant "dots" on their everyday maps.

Similar to chronic illness, experiences of social anxiety are invariably contingent on individual circumstances, environments and situations that cause experiences to rupture and flare but are, for the most part, invisible (Charmaz, 1995; Moss and Dyck, 2003). Samuels (2003, p. 248) argues that the focus on visibility by disability theorists "continues to render nonvisible disabilities invisible while reinforcing the exact cultural reliance on visibility that oppresses all of us". Samuels (2003) critiques the politics of visibility and the focus on physical markers of difference prevalent in theories of disability. The focus on the specular not only leads her to "question" whether she, living with a chronic, life-altering and invisible condition, "qualifies" as disabled, but it also limits our understanding of what disability is and further marginalises those whose social identities are un(der)recognised, called into question or disputed outright. To contextualise the "complexity and multiplicity of social restrictions" (Mulvany, 2000, p. 585) encountered by people experiencing mental and/or emotional distress, it is crucial to draw connections between the vaguely visible or invisible presentation of their experiences and their everyday use of space. Gail's narrative is particularly instructive:

> I found a website, "Disabled Travel Advice", when I was searching for information to help me get about with less anxiety. I don't know what I was expecting but it wasn't all that helpful. It said something like, ["Don't be shy about taking a seat at the front of the bus."] I could never, ever. I'm 33, I am physically able, you know? What a way to draw attention to myself! [...] Sitting on the bus isn't somewhere I want to start talking to someone at all, never mind about my mental health!
>
> (Gail, IR)

sitting in "priority seating" would provide her with a little more personal space and enable her to exit the bus more quickly alleviating some of Gail's anxieties, she is firmly attuned to the fact that she possesses no outward sign of impairment. Being young and "physically able", the socially and culturally "accepted markers" of disability are missing. The "solution" appears to present more problems than it solves, as sitting in priority seating areas is a perceived transgression of the social rules of public transport use. Furthermore, such a scenario could incite possible confrontation with others: Gail does not want to put herself in a position where she has to justify her use of the space and, by extension, her mental health. Arguably, the issue of (in)visibility presents further problems in terms of justification when "fraudulent" claims to space or "undeserving" accommodations are made (Lingsom, 2008) (also evident in the workplace, in Chapter 6). Gail's (IR) anticipated fears are similarly realised in Anna's (IR) experience:

> [I] sat in the disabled seats because the bus was really busy and I wanted to be able to get off if I needed to, you know? And an older woman called me out on it [...] She said I had no right to sit there [...] I got right off the bus [...] It really stuck with me. [Travelling is] difficult enough without being called out [on it].

Anna is one of few participants to discuss face-to-face confrontations in public spaces, and it is particularly poignant as she was challenged and publicly reprimanded for occupying "disabled spaces". Unfortunately, the experience has stayed with her, invariably influencing her perceptions and use of the public transport system as well as her "place" within it. Gail and Anna's experiences resonate with Thomas (2007) concept of "psycho-emotional dimensions of disability" that concerns the harmful words or actions of non-disabled people towards people with (non)visible impairments. Thomas (2007, p. 72) argues that "the damage inflicted works alongside psychological and emotional pathways, impacting negatively on self-esteem, personal confidence and ontological security", aspects that, for people with social anxiety, are already particularly low and vulnerable.

Sarah (QR) no longer travels by public transport as she frequently experiences panic attacks when in close proximity to other people. Commenting on the response of others to her episodes of panic, she writes: "people had no idea what to do, they would just stare like I was nuts or blatantly avoid getting involved". Cresswell argues that the "occurrence of out of place phenomena leads people to question behaviour and define what is and is not appropriate for a particular setting" (1996, p. 22). Here, Goffman's "aversion" takes on a different meaning, insofar as Sarah is the subject who is deemed "unworthy" of acknowledgement as her behaviour does not "fit" with the space. As such, she is rendered "out of place" and altogether ignored by her fellow commuters. Others also discussed perceived safety in terms of vulnerability and risk of becoming the target of harassment. Amanda states that "travelling home from work on the night bus with groups of drunk people in case they say something or try to get my attention" causes her incredible discomfort. Equally, Paul feels that he is an "easy target for young people to mock, looking and feeling so awkward that it draws their attention like I've got a big sign over me", leading him to avoid travel. Feminist geographers have argued that it is women's fear of crime, violence and harassment in the public sphere that overwhelmingly contributes to their decisions to avoid public transport (Valentine, 1989; Law, 1999). However, Day *et al.* (2003) further problematise gendered accounts of fear in public space, arguing that men's perceived vulnerability increases when they are placed in situations that are uncertain or unfamiliar, particularly where there is the potential for confrontation, as experienced by Paul, heightening his sense of negative expectation and further disrupting his relationship with the surrounding space. Whether these journeys are endured, altered or abandoned; new social routines, practices and negotiations unfold between home, work and social spheres of life in bringing about a sense of stability and to regain control over the self- and body-in-space. While the impact of their use is considerable, those who avoid public transport often walk considerable distances, rely heavily on family members or remain within the confines of the home (Chapter 6).

Concluding remarks

This chapter has demonstrated how sustained experiences of social anxiety play a significant role in regulating, restricting and, as suggested in the opening quotation, a shrinking social and spatial worlds (Dyck, 1995; Davidson, 2000;

Driedger, Crooks and Bennett, 2004). Throughout, this chapter has focused on the relation and embodied encounters between self-other-world highlighting the ways in which the "fine-grained" micro-textures of social space can trigger and sustain anxious experiences. Precarious and uncertain social and interpersonal worlds are compounded by an overwhelming fear of humiliation, embarrassment and rejection that has the potential to lead to an avoidance of social life and sustained experiences of isolation and loneliness. People's perceptions of social interactions and situations impact how they construct meaning from them, often exacerbating existing anxieties and fuelling new ones that shape their self-image, identity and ability to participate in, and contribute to, social worlds. A deeper examination of participant's social worlds uncovers the complexity in, and limitations placed on, everyday social life. Opportunities for encounter, both passing and sustained, become increasingly diminished, leading to further erosion of already restricted social and geographical worlds. Finally, I attend to the various ways everyday mobilities are disrupted and renegotiated in response to the temporally and spatially contingent nature of anxiety. Public space, for many participants, is full of intolerable disruptions to their daily geographies as individuals feel encumbered by uncertainty, perceived visibility, the potential for social interactions with others and the levels of social performance involved in, for example, buying a ticket or crossing the street. Consequently, social, spatial and temporal adjustments are made to the practice of everyday life that sees routes disrupted, journeys (re)negotiated and bodies (re)mobilised in creative but time-consuming ways.

Note

1 Grandmother.

References

Adey, P. (2017) *Mobility*. London: Routledge.
Bilecen, B. (2014) 'Friendship as "emotional work"', in B. Bilecen (ed.) *International Student Mobility and Transnational Friendships*. London: Palgrave Macmillan UK, pp. 51–70. https://doi.org/10.1057/9781137405258_3
Binnie, J. et al. (2007) 'Mundane mobilities, banal travels', *Social & Cultural Geography*, 8(2), pp. 165–174. https://doi.org/10.1080/14649360701360048
Bissell, D. (2007) 'Animating suspension: Waiting for mobilities', *Mobilities*, 2(2), pp. 277–298. https://doi.org/10.1080/17450100701381581
Bissell, D. (2010) 'Passenger mobilities: Affective atmospheres and the sociality of public transport', *Environment and Planning D: Society and Space*, 28(2), pp. 270–289. https://doi.org/10.1068/d3909
Bissell, D., Vannini, P. and Jensen, O.B. (2017) 'Intensities of mobility: Kinetic energy, commotion and qualities of supercommuting', *Mobilities*, 12(6), pp. 795–812. https://doi.org/10.1080/17450101.2016.1243935
Bondi, L. and Davidson, J. (2008) 'Situating gender', in L. Nelson and J. Seager (eds) *A Companion to Feminist Geography*. John Wiley & Sons.
Busfield, J. (2017) *Men, Women and Madness: Understanding Gender and Mental Disorder*. Bloomsbury Publishing.

Butterfield, A. and Martin, D. (2016) 'Affective sanctuaries: Understanding Maggie's as therapeutic landscapes', *Landscape Research*, 41(6), pp. 695–706. https://doi.org/1 0.1080/01426397.2016.1197386

Charmaz, K. (1995) 'The body, identity, and self', *Sociological Quarterly*, 36, pp. 657–680. https://doi.org/10.1111/j.1533-8525.1995.tb00459.x

Cresswell, T. (1996) *In Place/Out of Place: Geography, Ideology, and Transgression*. NED-New edition. Nebraska: University of Minnesota Press.

Davidson, J. (2000) '"… the world was getting smaller": Women, agoraphobia and bodily boundaries', *Area*, 32(1), pp. 31–40.

Davidson, J. (2001) 'Fear and trembling in the mall: Women, agoraphobia, and body boundaries', in Dycki, I., Davis Lewis, N., and McLafferty, S. (eds.) *Geographies of Women's Health*. London: Routledge, pp. 213–230.

Day, K., Stump, C. and Carreon, D. (2003) 'Confrontation and loss of control: Masculinity and men's fear in public space', *Journal of Environmental Psychology*, 23(3), pp. 311–322. https://doi.org/10.1016/S0272-4944(03)00024-0

Driedger, S.M., Crooks, V.A. and Bennett, D. (2004) 'Engaging in the disablement process over space and time: Narratives of persons with multiple sclerosis in Ottawa, Canada', *The Canadian Geographer / Le Géographe canadien*, 48(2), pp. 119–136. https://doi.org/10.1111/j.0008-3658.2004.00051.x

Dyck, I. (1995) 'Hidden geographies: The changing lifeworlds of women with multiple sclerosis', *Social Science & Medicine*, 40(3), pp. 307–320. https://doi.org/10.1016/0277-9536(94)E0091-6

Frie, R. (2017) 'Narratives of loneliness', in O. Sagan and E. Miller (eds) *Narratives of Loneliness: Multidisciplinary Perspectives from the 21st Century*. London: Routledge.

Giddens, A. (1991) *Modernity and Self-identity: Self and Society in the Late Modern Age*. Stanford University Press.

Glover, T.D. and Parry, D.C. (2009) 'A third place in the everyday lives of people living with cancer: Functions of Gilda's Club of Greater Toronto', *Health & Place*, 15(1), pp. 97–106. https://doi.org/10.1016/j.healthplace.2008.02.007

Goffman, E. (1971). *Relations in Public: Microstudies of the Public Order*. Basic Books

Hickinbottom-Brawn, S. (2013) 'Brand "you": The emergence of social anxiety disorder in the age of enterprise', *Theory & Psychology*, 23(6), pp. 732–751. https://doi.org/10.1177/0959354313500579

Hulme, M. and Truch, A. (2006). 'The role of interspace in sustaining identity', in P. Glotz, S. Bertschi, and C. Locke (eds) *Thumb Culture: The Meaning of Mobile Phones for Society*, pp. 137–148.

Imrie, R. (2000) 'Disability and discourses of mobility and movement', *Environment and Planning A: Economy and Space*, 32(9), pp. 1641–1656. https://doi.org/10.1068/a331

Jackson, P. and Everts, J. (2010) 'Anxiety as social practice', *Environment and Planning A: Economy and Space*, 42(11), pp. 2791–2806. https://doi.org/10.1068/a4385

Jeffres, L. et al. (2009) 'The impact of third places on community quality of life', *Applied Research in Quality of Life*, 4, pp. 333–345. https://doi.org/10.1007/s11482-009-9084-8

Laurier, E. and Philo, C. (2006) 'Possible geographies: A passing encounter in a café', *Area*, 38(4), pp. 353–363. https://doi.org/10.1111/j.1475-4762.2006.00712.x

Law, R. (1999) 'Beyond "women and transport": Towards new geographies of gender and daily mobility', *Progress in Human Geography*, 23(4), pp. 567–588. https://doi.org/10.1191/030913299666161864

Lingsom, S. (2008) 'Invisible impairments: Dilemmas of concealment and disclosure', *Scandinavian Journal of Disability Research*, 10(1), pp. 2–16. https://doi.org/10.1080/15017410701391567

Maslach, C. (1993) 'Burnout: A multidimensional perspective', in *Professional Burnout: Recent Developments in Theory and Research*, pp. 19–32. https://doi.org/10.4324/9781315227979-3

McCormack, D.P. (2008) 'Engineering affective atmospheres on the moving geographies of the 1897 Andrée expedition', *Cultural Geographies*, 15(4), pp. 413–430.

Moss, P. and Dyck, I. (2003) *Women, Body, Illness: Space and Identity in the Everyday Lives of Women with Chronic Illness*. Rowman & Littlefield Publishers.

Mulvany, J. (2000). 'Disability, impairment or illness? The relevance of the social model of disability to the study of mental disorder', *Sociology of Health & Illness*, 22, pp. 582–601. https://doi.org/10.1111/1467-9566.00221

NICE (2013) *Social anxiety disorder: Recognition, assessment and treatment*. Clinical guideline 159. National Institute for Health and Care Excellence, p. 37.

Oldenburg, R. (1999) *The Great Good Place: Cafes, Coffee Shops, Bookstores, Bars, Hair Salons, and Other Hangouts at the Heart of a Community*. New York: Hachette Books.

Olfson, M., Guardino, M., Struening, E., Schneier, F.R., Hellman, F., and Klein, D.F. (2000). 'Barriers to the treatment of social anxiety', *AJP*, 157, pp. 521–527. https://doi.org/10.1176/appi.ajp.157.4.521

Pahl, R. (2000) *On Friendship*. Wiley.

Parr, H. (2000) 'Interpreting the "hidden social geographies" of mental health: Ethnographies of inclusion and exclusion in semi-institutional places', *Health & Place*, 6(3), pp. 225–237. https://doi.org/10.1016/S1353-8292(00)00025-3

Samuels, E.J. (2003) 'My body, my closet: Invisible disability and the limits of coming-out discourse', *GLQ: A Journal of Lesbian and Gay Studies*, 9(1–2), pp. 233–255.

Smart, C. et al. (2012) 'Difficult friendships and ontological insecurity', *The Sociological Review*, 60(1), pp. 91–109. https://doi.org/10.1111/j.1467-954X.2011.02048.x

Southgate, K. (2016). *A Potential Space: Discovering a Place for D.W. Winnicott in the Psychoanalytic Literature on Drug Addiction (Psy.D.)* IL, USA: The Chicago School of Professional Psychology.

Thomas, C. (2007) *Sociologies of Disability and Illness: Contested Ideas in Disability Studies and Medical Sociology*. London: Macmillan Education UK.

Tough, H., Siegrist, J. and Fekete, C. (2017) 'Social relationships, mental health and wellbeing in physical disability: A systematic review', *BMC Public Health*, 17(1), p. 414. https://doi.org/10.1186/s12889-017-4308-6

Valentine, G. (1989) 'The geography of women's fear', *Area*, 21(4), pp. 385–390.

Weiss, R.S. (1973) *Loneliness: The experience of emotional and social isolation*. Cambridge: The MIT Press (Loneliness: The experience of emotional and social isolation), pp. xxii, 236.

Winnicott, D.W. (1971). *Playing and Reality*. Psychology Press.

Zimmerman, L. (1999) 'Public and potential space: Winnicott, Ellison, and Delillo', *The Centennial Review*, 43(3), pp. 565–574.

8 The (un)habitual geographies of social anxiety

Introduction

The "everydayness" of life is typically framed through the "unthinking" capacities of habit, a series of repeated and embodied practices and interactions so entrenched in our daily lives that they establish a tacit sense of familiarity and stability between a person and their socio-spatial worlds. This prevalent understanding of habit and the habitual largely ignores those people for whom such practices and interactions feature more pervasively in the navigation of social and spatial life, as well as the multitude of factors that impinge on a person's capacity to develop, maintain and ingrain habitual practices.

Drawing on a relational framework, social anxiety is defined as a "habit of fearful self-protection" that is entangled, on the one hand, with a "heightened state of anxious distress in the face of looming social threats" and, on the other, "the social or interpersonal environment within which the [anxious experience] is embedded" (Stravynski, 2014, p. 90). Pervasive patterns of social anxiety shape how individuals navigate their social and spatial worlds, disrupting habitual activities and interactions with and within them. While avoidant behaviours are common, many people endure social situations despite the intense levels of distress experienced, often with serious repercussions to their health and wellbeing (Stravynski, 2014). Consequently, individuals adopt a range of techniques to mitigate the intensities of their anxieties and manage the tensions, shifts and uncertainties of social space. These mitigation techniques are the empirical focus of this chapter.

Here I see how people embody and enact social anxiety within the context of habitual geographies (Bissell, 2013; Dewsbury and Bissell, 2015; Lea et al., 2015) by uncovering the practices and routines put in place as people adapt to interactions and events experienced as anxiety provoking and distressing. In order to understand the relational dynamics, I recognise the habitual presence of anxiety as a deeply unsettling and disruptive force, one that is innately entangled with, and embedded within, the spatialities and temporalities of everyday life. As a secondary aim, I contribute to existing theories of habit by reconfiguring habit as a set of practices that cannot embed seamlessly into everyday routine but, instead, are routinely written, un-written and re-written as individuals orient their social worlds.

DOI: 10.4324/9781003206880-8

Habit

The long and complex history of habit is well documented (Sparrow and Hutchinson, 2013). Contemporary approaches, particularly in the social sciences, influenced by Bourdieu's (1990) "habitus" and Merleau-Ponty's (2012) "embodied consciousness", designate a "unifying" and "integrative" capacity (Alexander, 1987, p. 147) enabling humans to encounter socio-spatial and material worlds unproblematically. Phenomenological considerations, integrating habit with discussions on embodiment, highlight the mutually co-constitutive relationship between body and world, one that is embodied and embedded in/through habitual practice (McGuirk 2014; Sheets-Johnstone, 2014). Habitus, an "embodied history", outlines the integration of past experiences as key to understanding how individuals respond to, and cope with, ever-changing conditions (Bourdieu, 1990). Collectively, these theoretical traditions have oriented geographical engagements with habit.

Habit is an important conceptual route for navigating the spatialities and temporalities of everyday life (Bissell, 2011; Dewsbury and Bissell, 2015; Seamon, 2015). The composition of social life, its structure and routine predictability, is built on the repetition of practice through which unreflective modes of being-in-the-world materialise. These dynamics play out within the backdrop of the unspoken routine and regularisation of everyday life, encoded in the essential pre-cognitive and pre-discursive articulations of self, body and world, thereby constituting an unreflective and habitually performed set of everyday practices and knowledge (Binnie et al. 2007, p. 165). Phenomenological concerns have focused on embodied habits, or "place-ballets" (Seamon, 1979, p. 55), to capture the rhythm and fluidity of everyday time-space and body routines. More recently, non-representational approaches have focused on the practices, events, relationships and affective resonances to capture how habits are embodied, embedded and emplaced (Thrift, 2008). The situated and intricate relationship between "internal" mental habits and "external" practice is reflected in the embodied geographies of everyday performance and mobility where through practices of walking and commuting (Edensor, 2003; Binnie *et al.*, 2007; Middleton, 2011); and corporeal experiences of movement and rest (Seamon, 2015), reliable rhythms ingrain a sense of stability and security in the practice of everyday life.

Others (notably Lea et al., 2015) seek to disrupt the reproductive nature through which habitual life is considered to emerge. Through the vein of mindful meditation, Lea et al. (2015) explore how mindful practice cultivates awareness of automatic thoughts, feelings and actions. Crucially, this practice is not in an attempt to transform the whole self but to acknowledge the relationship *with* the self, one that advocates a non-judgemental, conscious reflection on the relationship with existing habits. Interestingly, they focus on habit as both a set of individual practices and one embedded within wider socio-cultural and material contexts. In doing so, they address how particular practices *become* routinised as habit and consider the "*process* through which we gain sense, understanding and awareness" (Dewsbury and Bissell, 2015, p. 26) of existing habits.

Overwhelmingly, engagements with habit in geography and beyond have overstated the ease with which habitual and routine forms of action become ingrained and play out in day-to-day life particularly as much of the existing research reflects an assumed synchronicity between body and world that is not accessible to all.

The disruption of everyday life

The habitual nature of everyday life often comes sharply into view when something happens to destabilise established and ingrained routines. Experiences of health, illness and disability disrupt the apparent synchronicity and fluidity that routine and ritualised aspects of everyday life are said to engender. In these contexts, everyday habits, including routines and mobilities (physical, social or otherwise), may be affected, limited and/or restricted (Chouinard, 1999; Moss and Dyck, 2003). The onset of chronic illness has the capacity to disrupt life-long habits while necessitating new routines are established to help stabilise health and wellbeing. Habitual actions and routines are vulnerable to unpredictable states of being as lives are/become "temporally dynamic" and "routinely unpredictable" (Crooks, 2010, p. 59). Smith (2012), providing insight into how "non-conforming" bodies unsettle taken-for-granted spaces and activities through lived experiences of epilepsy, questions the extent to which individuals become habituated to living with the uncertainty and unpredictability of seizures. The relatively unpredictable nature of the epileptic body renders social space inherently unpredictable, wherein "[r]outines once taken-for-granted are deliberately discontinued or forcibly altered to accommodate potential losses of control" (2012, p. 351).

The embodied reality of disability adjusts the lens of what is or can be considered to be(come) habitual. Engman and Cranford (2016) argue that existing theories on habit have neglected to take into account non-normative bodies and behaviours in the development and maintenance of habits. They highlight how disabled people adapt and make adjustments to socio-spatial and material environments that are "preconfigured" for normative bodies. Physical, social and systemic barriers render habits "perpetually suspended in a space of precarity" (Engman and Cranford, 2016, p. 38) as they involve considerable amounts of energy and emotional labour to manage. Similarly, acknowledging the "timings and spacings" of everyday life of disability, Hansen and Philo (2007, p. 497) contend that the practices of daily living are habitual only in the sense that they are practised within the context of everyday life, and that the "time, space and speed realities" of carrying out tasks for many disabled people require strategic negotiation and microscopic planning.

Collectively, these studies have paid significant attention to the ways in which various health and/or embodied experiences disrupt daily routines, times and spaces, but they have largely avoided an *explicit* engagement with theories of habit (exceptions: Rowles, 2000; Lea, Cadman and Philo, 2015). Existing theories of habit focus on the capacity of people to mould into normative temporalities and spatialities; thus, it is imperative that habit is reconfigured to acknowledge and include the day-to-day consequences of health, illness and disability as chronic, fluctuating, long-term and/or life-long experiences, through which habitualised ways of living are disrupted, mitigated, adapted and re-established. There is a need, again, in human geography "to see habits and routines afresh" (Rose, 1993, p. 46).

(Un)habitual geographies of social anxiety

Social anxiety is a thoroughly embodied experience with habits of mind and body fuelling anxious experiences. Enduring cycles of rumination and anticipation (Chapter 4) play a fundamental role in this relationship wherein, habits of mind, "spurred by expectations" of social interactions, are animated and exacerbated by the "felt dynamic of apprehension" through the body (Sheets-Johnstone, 2014). Crucially, this raises questions about to what extent do the bodily dynamics of anxiety, fear and apprehension, which serve to embolden anxious experiences, disrupt our habitual understanding of habit. Anderson's (2010, p. 777) "anticipatory action" advocates that geographies are "made and lived in the name of pre-empting, preparing for, or preventing threats"; although originally applied in the context of threats to liberal democracies, such actions are no less relevant in this instance. Anticipatory processes capture how past experiences are projected into the future, and thus shaping the practices, itineraries and routines of the present. Such anticipatory notions are deeply intertwined with understandings of the habitual: on the one hand, they set in motion the transformative potential of habitual practices and routines that establish control and predictability; on the other, they embody the immanent and foreboding disruptive capacity of uncertainty, highlighting the temporal and spatial complexity of living with social anxiety.

Such affective dimensions of experience mark the "emergence of unpredictability" (Grosz, 2013, p. 225), unhinging the very "illusion of consistency" (Bissell, 2010, p. 85) that the habitual practice of everyday life intends to cement. Bissell (2009) discusses the affective forces that press upon the chronically pained body, drawing attention to the complexities of intensity to consider the relational capacity of the body and those experiences that "take place during spatially and temporally distributed encounters" (Anderson, 2006, p. 735). In social anxiety, the viscerality of experience embodied in symptomatic warning signs not only give rise to a heightened sense of self and bodily awareness that becomes "sensorially overwhelming, emotionally uncomfortable, socially stigmatising and so, *disabling*" (Davidson and Parr, 2010, p. 63), but also to a heightened sense of being visible and, by extension, exposed to potential scrutiny by others – similar to experiences of agoraphobia (Davidson, 2003).

What becomes apparent, then, is the habitual pattern of anxiety, which can be articulated in two interrelated ways: first, a self-reflexive practice (Lea et al., 2015) which, I would argue, is habitually self-critical, manifesting in highly negative views of self and a painful and repetitive self-scrutiny, characterised by harsh internal dialogues about social performance or perceived failures. Social interactions and encounters are then performed, re-performed, re-played and ruminated over in excruciatingly minute detail, generating anxiety-drenched anticipations which increase in intensity about what could go wrong in future settings. This disruptive embodied temporality suggests the non-linear experience of time through which socially anxious experience emerges, with both past and future impinging on present activity (Chapter 4). Second, as an affective force that mobilises and amplifies one's awareness of, and experience in, their socio-spatial environments. By concentrating on experiential accounts, this exploration of social anxiety illustrates how individuals actively use space and specific strategies to regain control of their bodies and surroundings in order to manage everyday beings and doings that are tainted by pervasive anxieties and uncertainties. In this sense, the anxious body is *moved* by perceptions and affections into *motion* through movement and action (Fuchs and Koch, 2014).

Managing time and space

In order to limit the uncertainty of daily life, participants engage in the strategic planning of space-time routines and movements in an anticipatory and preventative vein of micro-managing potential embarrassing and humiliating encounters *out* of the interactions, situations and events that constitute everyday life. It requires implementing routinised practices of living and a strict timetabling of time and space, seeking to ensure minimal disruption to the carrying out of everyday tasks. Thereby enabling managed involvement in particular spheres of everyday life or within particular spaces that individuals find difficult to negotiate:

> I need to know what is going on in my day, I like to have a timetable and I like to know exactly what time I need to get there and exactly what time I need to leave. If I go places I haven't been before and don't know what to expect I'll have a panic attack. So, I'll research a place online before I go or look for advice on how to do something, plan it out, write some notes and run through it in my head so I don't make a mistake or look stupid. I've just got to keep myself together.
>
> (Natalie, IR)

Natalie's practice of time-tabling is implemented in a bid to reduce external interferences by allocating specific time restrictions on daily tasks, as well as furnishing herself with enough knowledge to reduce the unexpected. Reflective of Anderson's (2010) "anticipatory action", wherein unknown futures are imagined and enacted upon, she acknowledges the significance of being able to map places out beforehand in order to "get a feel for a place" that is unfamiliar. She draws attention to some of the difficulties that cause her anxieties to arise

– how others perceive her, appearing "stupid", or not doing something in the correct way – and demonstrates how she manages her behaviours by research-ing, planning and rehearsing social interactions (McGrath, Reavey and Brown, 2008). Elsewhere, she notes that this rehearsal can "cement" her *in*ability to do something rather than providing the momentum to carry it through. The habitual exposure and repetition has the potential to keep her in a state of high alert, as opposed to cementing the practice into an everyday routine.

The unpredictable nature of social space is emphasised further. There is less of a seamless and fluid choreography between self and world and more of a series of sharp and repetitive transitions as a person navigates daily life. Spaces between destinations are strategically negotiated since simply getting from A to B may be(come) difficult if the threat of interactions or the intensity of her surrounding space increases (Dyck, 1995). Structuring a strict routine into everyday life also places limitations on daily tasks so that Natalie does not become overwhelmed. This strategic planning highlights an intolerance of uncertainty, and, while extending control over the temporal and spatial dimen-sions of experience, is ultimately a process of creating, or maintaining, a cohe-sive, bounded and functional sense of self: indeed, an act of "keeping herself together".

Spatial routes

Participants describe how they use and move through space at particular times and in particular ways. For many, social space is constantly changing in terms of intensity, even in known and familiar environments. As such, individuals do not move through space passively or unreflexively, for there is usually an active, ongoing re-negotiating of their socio-spatial surroundings:

> Say I'm going to the shops; I'll take a longer, quieter route. I could walk in about 10 minutes, it's a straight road through the main street but there's pubs with people smoking outside I need to walk past and it's generally busy, cars and crossings, there's usually always someone who knows you and wants to stop and chat and I just can't, it's too much. Even just hav-ing those people look at me or if I make eye contact with them, it's too much.
>
> (Lara, IR)

Sheets-Johnstone (2014, p. 98) argues that habit is about "have made the strange familiar" but arguably, for Lara, the familiar is equally intolerable. It is apparent that completing everyday tasks is intensely marked by layers of potential interaction with other people and objects. These components of everyday social space become obstacles to her being able to move uncon-strained by anxiety due to intensely anticipated interactions. Particular envi-ronments, or even the process of getting to particular places, are laced with specific anxieties provoking a sensory tension which becomes "too much" for her to cope with. Her experiences are illustrative of the 55% of questionnaire respondents who feel "unsafe" or "very unsafe" in busy streets. Equipped with knowledge of the local environment and anticipating distressing encounters, Lara practices specific spatial mobilities where she "re-routes" her journey, enabling a level of control to be extended over her socio-spatial surroundings and, by extension, the palpable signals of her anxiety. She continues:

> I go early and go along the river where it is quiet. It probably triples the length of my journey, but it keeps my anxiety down and it's quieter [with] less people, I'm constantly on guard for people who might run by or come onto the path but I can usually get myself in a good head-space for doing what I need to do that day.
>
> (Lara, IR)

Taking into account the temporal and spatial adjustments made to Lara's journey, by choosing particular times and routes that are quieter, we see how these anticipatory moves cause space to be used and re-negotiated in order to "strategically intervene on the future" (Anderson, 2010, p. 785). Lara also notes that if she "feels" like something unexpected will happen, she "might vere off [course]". Her daily mobilities rarely "unfold" on "auto-pilot" (Middleton, 2011, p. 2874) as she still remains attuned to her surroundings, aware that they cannot be completely certain or known. The habitual dimensions present in these everyday movements emerge through pre-empting the difficulties that she may face. However, altering her daily routes also affords her the mental time and space to prepare for the day ahead and take preventative measures against an anxiety attack.

Donna reports similar feelings about walking in public:

> I get incredibly anxious walking down the street and become so self-conscious about myself, how I'm walking or drawing any attention to myself whatsoever. It's so awful and unpredictable. Crossing the road can be absolute hell. All the cars are stopped at the lights and I feel like I'm being glared at [...] I don't go out much but if I need to I plan, plan, plan and won't leave the house when I know it will be mayhem outside.
>
> (Donna, IR)

Donna's experience marks a clear boundary between the feelings of uncertainty associated with external social space and the feelings of safety and security engendered by being at home. Similar to Lara, she places specific emphasis on planning and completely avoids situations and spaces that she knows will be detrimental to her social wellbeing. These obstacles uncover something of the "hidden geographies" (Dyck, 1995) of social anxiety in which it is evident how the micro-textures, the unthinking practice of walking and crossing the road, create and sustain a crippling self-consciousness and palpable awareness of the occupation of social space.

For similar reasons, others favour going outside at night. Craig notes that "night walks" are a "huge coping strategy" for him:

> Every couple of nights I'll go a walk, especially if I'm feeling cooped up. I feel so much better about going out when it's dark outside. I'm less likely to cross paths with anyone but even if I do I've got my hat on and a hood up so no one is going to speak to me.
>
> (Craig, QR)

Craig also notes, "but I'm a guy so...", in reference to the feelings of safety he has while walking alone at night, a feeling and reality which is often not afforded to women (Valentine, 1989).

Spatial screens

Objects, clothing and (trusted) people are also used as protective barriers between the self and other people when in public. Karen's social anxieties are centred on being visible to, and approached by, other people. She rarely leaves the perceived safety of her home except to attend routine appointments with her doctor or therapist, stating:

> I get taxis everywhere. Literally, I go in with my sunglasses on and block out the whole world and my mum comes with me – everywhere I go my mum comes with me because I'm so terrified.
>
> (Karen, IR)

Karen implements a number of self-protection strategies including travelling only when accompanied by her mother and using taxis for very short journeys (e.g. less than five minutes to her local health centre). Although still incredibly restricted by her anxieties, these are small ways in which she improves her limited daily mobility so as not to be rendered entirely housebound (Law, 1999). Crucially, her mother operates as a barrier between her and any unexpected social contact limiting her involvement (and expectations to "perform") in the social and exposure to perceived threats (Davidson, 2003). Similar themes emerged among other participants, who convey the feelings of protection engineered by wearing sunglasses:

> [W]hen I do go out, I wear sunglasses and my anxiety is significantly less severe, like I'm protected. I'm not as exposed as there is always this barrier between me and the outside world [...] especially if there's an occasion I need to speak to someone, I don't obsess about whether I was making too little or too much eye contact and what they must have thought of me.
>
> (Anya, QR)

Sunglasses hence operate as a social shield between the anxious self and the invasive gaze of others (Davidson, 2003). This perceived visibility renders the subject "under surveillance" leaving them open to ridicule, judgement and scrutiny by others about their (in)ability to perform "correctly" in social space. The gaze operates as an "invasion" as "social space threatens to become corrosive rather than constitutive of our identities" (Davidson, 2003, 120). Pointing to the intricacies that provoke her anxiety, Anya finds the uncertainty of social space particularly invasive. Being "under surveillance" is an intensely *felt* experience that is inherently tied to notions of social performance and behaviour and how she believes she is perceived by others. Anya's story is instructive of how "habitual patterns of thought transform what might otherwise be a fleeting negative feeling/thought into a more enduring form of negativity or rumination" (Lea et al., 2015, p. 55) through her tendency to "obsess", reflect and ruminate over the microscopic details of social encounters.

Other objects such as clothing, to not "draw any attention to myself" (Clare, QR), and earphones/headphones, "to isolate myself" (Lauren, QR), are also used in public spaces:

Clothes are a big security blanket, I tend to wear very plain, long and loose fitted clothing. No brands or slogans or anything like that. Cardigans, jumpers, long t-shirts. Minimal make up. Plain Jane!

Frith and Gleeson (2008, p. 256) discuss the relationship between body image and clothing practices, noting that clothes are used as a strategy to conceal "the size, shape or appearance of the body", in Clare's case it is used to conceal the presence of her body: "I just don't want anyone to notice me or draw attention to me in any way whatsoever!". There is also a practical element to wearing loose clothing especially as Claire notes she is prone to "overheating and sweating whenever I'm in public". Lauren discusses wearing earphones to similar ends:

I've always got earphones in all the time. If I need to go anywhere or do anything I'll listen to music or an audio book to help keep me calm and focused on what I need to do, or if I find my anxiety really ramping up I'll listen to a guided meditation. I always make sure they are visible too just so no one attempts to talk to me, just to ward them off a little, you know?

(Lauren, IR)

By wearing sunglasses, she feels less susceptible to the scrutiny and judgements to which she would otherwise feel "exposed" in encounters with other people, reducing the critical self-reflexivity lingering in the aftermath of an event. Both Karen and Anya's use of sunglasses, Clare's use of clothing and Lauren's use of earbuds as spatial screens highlight the intensity experienced in the perception of being visible to, or in the proximity of, other people, and revealing how the consequences of being seen become embodied in feelings of terror and exposure.

Moments of escape

The potential of what *could* go wrong in particular settings and environments is a central anticipatory concern of social anxiety experience and so people plan accordingly. However, once people are *in* social spaces, their social anxieties must be carefully managed and navigated. Fifty-three per cent of questionnaire respondents stated that they felt either "unsafe" or "very unsafe" in places of leisure such as restaurants or bars. This lack of safety is usually provoked by proximity to other people, atmospheric concerns about frenetic environments or those that become "too intense", and perceived pressures integral to placing an order, eating and drinking in front of others and asking for the bill. Despite these anxieties, individuals often endure social situations that have the potential to be(come) distressing and use their environments creatively to secure small moments of escape:

> If I'm forced into social situations I usually need to decompress every 20-25 mins or so XD[1] take a time out sort of thing. Go to the bathroom, pretend that I've forgotten something in the car, go outside for a smoke (once other folk have come back hahaha)
>
> (Alan, IR)

Nina notes that she performs an assessment of her immediate surroundings, usually mapping out safe(r) spaces within and situating herself next to potential escape routes:

> In a bar or restaurant I will immediately assess where the toilets and/or exits are so I can escape […] I never feel particularly comfortable [because] there's always too much going on around me.
>
> (Nina, IR)

She continues:

> I will always sit by a door for a quick escape if it got too intense or I'd use the toilet as a place to calm myself. I can go into a cubicle and have a breather and some privacy. Nobody knows I'm doing it because everybody goes to the toilet, so it wouldn't be seen as out of the ordinary.

The significance of toilets for participants as a temporary holding space was striking. Monica describes them as a "check point" that she can "duck in and out of" and Alan as a "sanctuary". The common notion of the toilet as a "dirty space" is here juxtaposed against its almost quasi-therapeutic nature. It should be noted that toilet spaces, particularly public toilets, did not always engender such feelings of safety for other participants. For some, these spaces entailed a very specific set of social anxieties about sharing space in close proximity to others, as well as also shame regarding bathroom behaviours and bodily processes, for example, being seen, heard or smelled (Barcan, 2010). Nonetheless, it enables Nina to contain herself within the boundaries of the cubicle to regain a sense of bodily and spatial control, echoing Longhurst's (2001, p. 66) assessment that toilets operate "as spaces in which bodies are (re)made and (re)sealed ready for public scrunity". Longhurst's comments resonate with the experiences of participants who are often finely attuned to, and anxious about, how they are perceived by other people. It also highlights the temporary nature of this "re-sealing" whereby, once Nina re-engages with the wider social environment, her anxieties are likely to re-emerge. Furthermore, the toilet operates as a space where her privacy is maintained, her (anxious) identity is protected, and her practices and behaviours are normalised.

These extracts illustrate a managed involvement in everyday life involving "invisible, embodied practical, emotional and social work" (Bell, Tyrrell and Phoenix, 2016, p. 184). This hidden work is as constraining as it is liberating in terms of the amount of time and the levels of preparation and rehearsal individuals invest. Carefully considered routines and practices often play out in a preventative vein and are adapted in response to events and interactions namely to "stop the effects of an event disrupting the circulations and interdependencies that make up a valued life" (Anderson, 2010, p. 791).

Concluding remarks

What becomes evident through these anxious subjectivities is the capacity of various social experiences and intensities of health to rupture habitual modes of being wherein particular encounters with other people and spaces are simultaneously experienced as familiar and distressing; routinely occurring, yet, disruptive. As such, these routines do not echo the *unreflexive* sentiments present in the habitual practice of everyday life (Edensor, 2007, p. 202) in which "regular routes are followed unquestioningly, all habits are rarely disrupted [and] where familiar space is consistently reproduced". Instead, they are jarred against an assemblage of anticipated encounters, spaces, objects and atmospheric and bodily affects. They are continually assessed and restructured in response to internal and symptomatic warning signs and various socio-spatial cues and clues. By exploring the day-to-day consequences of living with social anxiety this chapter complements existing research on disruptive experiences of mental and emotional health (Davidson, 2003; Parr, 1999; Segrott and Doel, 2004) and chronic illness and impairment (Crooks, 2007; Dyck, 1995; Lucherini, 2016; Smith, 2012) by paying attention to how participants experience and negotiate social anxiety (whether socially, spatially or otherwise) in the context of their everyday lives. Comparatively, attention needs to be paid to the disruptions caused to "whole" lives and the impact of wider ill-health trajectories on, for example, social lives, educational attainment and employment opportunities (Bell, Tyrrell and Phoenix, 2016).

Drawing on lived accounts of social anxiety, this chapter has explored those people for whom very little can become ingrained or goes unnoticed in the practice of everyday life but is always there, central to conscious self-reflection and a constant questioning of the self. Thus, life is never seamlessly habituated, but is, instead, constantly interrupted and re-visited. In doing so, it has unearthed a tension in how habit is conceptualised, where the very essence of habit exists

> somewhere between the necessity of ease and the torment of need, one side directed to making the world readily habitable, and making the living being at home in the familiar; the other directed to a trajectory of infinite repetition, a tic, an addiction, a limitation and constraint on life.
>
> (Grosz, 2013, p. 202)

If there is to be a sense of "habit" in the context of social anxiety, then it is in the specific assemblages where so many distressing and uncertain possibilities coalesce; manifest in the internal and external interferences, affective viscerality and the persistent rumination and anticipation that are so emblematic of social anxiety. What requires greater attention is the ways in which these intensities linger in the repetitive reflection upon the micro-textures of everyday life, where individuals are so often reliving past interactions in minute details. The exhaustive anticipation of future events – where the possibilities of what could go wrong viewed through the lens of negatively perceived past experiences – is considered routine and is evident in the strategic micro-planning enacted to circumvent potentially damaging events and interactions.

The focus on routines and practices fostered in response to the unpredictable nature of participants' socio-spatial surroundings illustrates how negotiating the intricacies of various interactions, situations, movements and encounters habitually experienced as distressing takes a substantial effort which may have long-term consequence for physical, mental and emotional wellbeing (Hansen and Philo, 2007). While much work remains to be done that incorporates lived accounts of social anxiety, this chapter provides insights into the ways in which people actively live with their social anxieties through painstakingly detailed, temporally and spatially specific practices that convey the pervasive and disruptive nature of their experiences; habitually unmaking and re-making the habits of a "normal" lifetime.

Acknowledgement

A version of this chapter was published previously as Boyle, L.E. (2019) The (un)habitual geographies of Social Anxiety Disorder, Social Science and Medicine, Special Issue "Hopeful adaptation" in health geographies: Seeking health and wellbeing in times of adversity, Vol. 231, pp. 31–37. It has been adapted for publication here in accordance with Elsevier re-use and copyright guidelines.

Note

1 "XD" is used to symbolise a laughing face. "X" symbolises a person's eyes squeezed shut and "D" represents a laughing mouth. Here it is in response to the frequency of Alan's "social breaks".

References

Alexander, T.M. (1987) *John Dewey's Theory of Art, Experience, and Nature: The Horizons of Feeling.* Albany, NY: SUNY Press.

Anderson, B. (2006) 'Becoming and being hopeful: Towards a theory of affect', *Environment and Planning D: Society and Space*, 24(5), pp. 733–752. https://doi.org/10.1068/d393t

Anderson, B. (2010) 'Preemption, precaution, preparedness: Anticipatory action and future geographies', *Progress in Human Geography*, 34(6), pp. 777–798. https://doi.org/10.1177/0309132510362600

Barcan, R. (2010) 'Dirty spaces: Separation, concealment, and shame in the public toilet', in M. Harvey and L. Noren (eds) *Toilet: Public Restrooms and the Politics of Sharing.* New York: NYU Press, pp. 25–46.

Bell, S.L., Tyrrell, J., and Phoenix, C. (2016) 'Ménière's disease and biographical disruption: Where family transitions collide', *Social Science & Medicine*, 166, pp. 177–185. https://doi.org/10.1016/j.socscimed.2016.08.025

Binnie, J. et al. (2007) 'Mundane mobilities, banal travels', *Social & Cultural Geography*, 8(2), pp. 165–174. https://doi.org/10.1080/14649360701360048

Bissell, D. (2009) 'Obdurate pains, transient intensities: Affect and the chronically pained body', *Environment and Planning A*, 41(4), pp. 911–928. https://doi.org/10.1068/a40309

Bissell, D. (2010) 'Placing affective relations: Uncertain geographies of pain', in B. Anderson and P. Harrison (eds) *Taking-Place: Non-Representational Theories and Geography.* Farnham: Ashgate, pp. 79–98.

Bissell, D. (2011) 'Thinking habits for uncertain subjects: Movement, stillness, susceptibility', *Environment and Planning A*, 43(11), pp. 2649–2665. https://doi.org/10.1068/a43589

Bissell, D. (2013) 'Habit displaced: The disruption of skilful performance', *Geographical Research*, 51(2), pp. 120–129. https://doi.org/10.1111/j.1745-5871.2012.00765.x

Bourdieu, P., 1990. *The Logic of Practice.* Stanford University Press.

Chouinard, V. (1999) 'Body politics: Disabled women's activism in Canada and beyond', in R. Butler and H. Parr (eds) *Mind and Body Spaces: Geographies of Illness, Impairment and Disability.* London: Routledge, pp. 269–296.

Crooks, V.A. (2007) 'Exploring the altered daily geographies and lifeworlds of women living with fibromyalgia syndrome: A mixed-method approach', *Social Science and Medicine*, 64(3), pp. 577–588.

Crooks, V.A. (2010) 'Women's changing experiences of the home and life inside it after becoming chronically ill', in *Towards Enabling Geographies: 'Disabled' Bodies and Minds in Society and Space.* Aldershot and Vermont: Ashgate Publishing, pp. 45–62.

Davidson, J. (2003) "'Putting on a face': Sartre, Goffman, and agoraphobic anxiety in social space', *Environment and Planning D: Society and Space*, 21(1), pp. 107–122.

Davidson, J. and Parr, H. (2010) 'Enabling cultures of dis/order online', in V. Chouinard, E. Hall, and R. Wilton (eds) *Towards Enabling Geographies: 'Disabled' Bodies and Minds in Society and Space*. Aldershot and Vermont: Ashgate Publishing, pp. 63–84.

Dewsbury, J.D. and Bissell, D. (2015) 'Habit geographies: the perilous zones in the life of the individual', *Cultural Geographies*, 22(1), pp. 21–28. https://doi.org/10.1177/1474474014561172

Dyck, I. (1995) 'Hidden geographies: The changing lifeworlds of women with multiple sclerosis', *Social Science and Medicine*, 40(3), pp. 307–320.

Edensor, T. (2003) 'Defamiliarizing the mundane roadscape', *Space and Culture*, 6(2), pp. 151–168. https://doi.org/10.1177/1206331203251257

Edensor, T. (2007) 'Mundane mobilities, performances and spaces of tourism', *Social & Cultural Geography*, 8(2), pp. 199–215. https://doi.org/10.1080/14649360701360089

Engman, A. and Cranford, C. (2016) 'Habit and the body: Lessons for social theories of habit from the experiences of people with physical disabilities', *Sociological Theory*, 34(1), pp. 27–44.

Frith, H. and Gleeson, K. (2008) 'Dressing the body: The role of clothing in sustaining body pride and Managing body distress', *Qualitative Research in Psychology*, 5(4), pp. 249–264. https://doi.org/10.1080/14780880701752950

Fuchs, T. and Koch, S.C. (2014) 'Embodied affectivity: On moving and being moved', *Frontiers in Psychology*, 5, p. 508. https://doi.org/10.3389/fpsyg.2014.00508

Grosz, E. (2013) 'Habit today: Ravaisson, Bergson, Deleuze and us', *Body & Society*, 19(2–3), pp. 217–239. https://doi.org/10.1177/1357034X12472544

Hansen, N. and Philo, C. (2007) 'The normality of doing things differently: Bodies, spaces and disability geography', *Tijdschrift voor economische en sociale geografie*, 98(4), pp. 493–506. https://doi.org/10.1111/j.1467-9663.2007.00417.x

Law, R. (1999) 'Beyond "women and transport": Towards new geographies of gender and daily mobility', *Progress in Human Geography*, 23(4), pp. 567–588. https://doi.org/10.1191/030913299666161864

Lea, J., Cadman, L. and Philo, C. (2015) 'Changing the habits of a lifetime? Mindfulness meditation and habitual geographies', *Cultural geographies*, 22(1), pp. 49–65. https://doi.org/10.1177/1474474014536519

Longhurst, R. (2001) *Bodies: Exploring Fluid Boundaries*. Psychology Press.

Lucherini, M. (2016) 'Performing diabetes: Surveillance and self-management', *Surveillance & Society*, 14(2), pp. 259–276.

McGrath, L., Reavey, P. and Brown, S.D. (2008) 'The scenes and spaces of anxiety: Embodied expressions of distress in public and private fora', *Emotion, Space and Society*, 1(1), pp. 56–64.

McGuirk, J. (2014) 'Phenomenological considerations of habit: Reason, knowing and self-presence in habitual action', *Phenomenology and Mind*, (6), pp. 112–121.

Merleau-Ponty, M. (2012) *Phenomenology of Perception*. Routledge.

Middleton, J. (2011) '"I'm on autopilot, I just follow the route": Exploring the habits, routines, and decision-making practices of everyday urban mobilities', *Environment and Planning A*, 43(12), pp. 2857–2877. https://doi.org/10.1068/a43600

Moss, P. and Dyck, I. (2003) *Women, Body, Illness: Space and Identity in the Everyday Lives of Women with Chronic Illness*. Rowman & Littlefield Publishers.

Parr, H. (1999) 'Delusional geographies: The experiential worlds of people during madness/illness', *Environment and Planning D: Society and Space*, 17(6), pp. 673–690.

Rose, G. (1993) *Feminism & Geography: The Limits of Geographical Knowledge*. Minneapolis, MN: U of Minnesota Press.

Rowles, G.D. (2000) 'Habituation and being in place', *The Occupational Therapy Journal of Research*, 20(1_suppl), pp. 52S–67S. https://doi.org/10.1177/15394492000200S105

Seamon, D. (1979) A geography of the lifeworld: movement, rest and encounter.

Seamon, D. (2015) *A Geography of the Lifeworld (Routledge Revivals): Movement, Rest and Encounter*. London: Routledge.

Segrott, J. and Doel, M.A. (2004) 'Disturbing geography: Obsessive-compulsive disorder as spatial practice', *Social & Cultural Geography*, 5(4), pp. 597–614.

Sheets-Johnstone, M. (2014) 'On the origin, nature, and genesis of habit', *Phenomenology and Mind*, pp. 76–89. https://doi.org/10.13128/Phe_Mi-19553

Smith, N. (2012) 'Embodying brainstorms: The experiential geographies of living with epilepsy', *Social & Cultural Geography*, 13(4), pp. 339–359.

Sparrow, T. and Hutchinson, A. (2013) *A History of Habit: From Aristotle to Bourdieu*. Lanham, MD: Lexington Books.

Stravynski, A. (2014) *Social Phobia: An Interpersonal Approach*. Cambridge: Cambridge University Press.

Thrift, N. (2008) *Non-Representational Theory: Space, Politics, Affect*. London: Routledge.

Valentine, G. (1989) 'The geography of women's fear', *Area*, 21(4), pp. 385–390.

9 Towards anxious geographies

This book is an examination of the personal geographies of living with social anxiety. Through a human geographical lens, this book situates social anxiety as a social and spatial phenomenon by analysing the spatialities, temporalities and embodiments of the anxious experience. This concluding chapter shifts its focus from the qualitative heart of the book towards a consideration of its primary arguments and contributions, points to avenues for future research, discusses some implications for policy and practice and finally, offers some closing thoughts on the unsung impacts of researching the people's anxious worlds.

Reimagining social anxiety

In many ways, social anxiety remains the neglected "disorder" that it was declared to be by Liebowitz and colleagues nearly 40 years ago, but not *only* in its offerings as a "fertile area of psychobiological and clinical investigation" (Liebowitz *et al.*, 1985, p. 729). Indeed, what has arguably been *more* palpably neglected by the reigning orthodoxies is the subjective experience of anxious distress, inclusive of the social fears and adversities that people with social anxiety face; the social, relational and embodied dynamics that enable and sustain the condition; and the different meanings that people find in, and ascribe to, the varied and grounded experiences of being socially anxious. Social anxiety, like many forms of emotional distress, is caught in a tension between, even restrained by, the dominant models that frame our understanding of it and for which the only available recourse is the "diagnostic gaze and therapeutic interventions of psychiatry" (Rose, 2006, p. 475). Alternative perspectives, particularly those questioning social anxiety's continued medicalisation, explain it either as a consequence of particular stresses and societal processes in our "postmodern" age or re-situate it alongside related concepts of shyness and embarrassment (Chapter 2).

One of the primary aims of this book has been to challenge and offer an alternative to the idea that the only lens that can adequately account for and recognise social anxiety is a biomedical one and lays a foundation for viewing social anxiety through a social and spatial lens. This leads from the position that purely "brain-based" assessments of social anxiety – that being those rooted in

DOI: 10.4324/9781003206880-9

the "functions of the cerebral architecture of individuals" (Fitzgerald and Callard, 2015, p. 7) and explained as manifestations of genetic and neurobiological abnormalities – are superficial, reductionist and overly simplistic explanatory frameworks through which to attend to complex social and existential states (Deacon, 2013; Deacon and McKay, 2015). Crucially, this does not intend to render the brain, or indeed the embodied symptoms of anxiety, obsolete, only to challenge the idea that social anxiety – inclusive of its associated thoughts, feelings, symptoms and behaviours – is reducible to it. As Pilgrim argues, "the brain affords our capacity to think, feel and act as human agents in contingent contexts but cannot ultimately explain any of these" (2020, p. 1). Equally, this is not a wholesale dismissal of the utility or value many find in a "diagnosis" of social anxiety but rather a prompt to cultivate a deeper understanding of how such categories and classifications operate in and shape people's lives, attending to how they become anxious and come to view themselves as such in line with particular biomedical models (or not). In light of this, Chapter 5 unpacks these aspects by exploring how biomedical accounts of social anxiety are situated alongside more personal and sociological explanations of distress and how this distinction feeds into different practices of, and modes of relating to, diagnosis.

This research has also involved attending to those experiences and expressions held firmly in the grasp of medicalised perspectives rather than ignoring them entirely for fear of "reinforcing" those models. This perspective includes, but is not limited to, reconceptualising "irrational" thoughts and beliefs, embodied physical symptoms and enacted behaviours as acquired and evolved responses to hostile and threatening social situations. However, as Johnstone and Boyle argue, care has to be taken that these aspects are not simply "assimilated back into individualistic accounts of emotional and psychological distress" (2020, p. 189). This book contributes to these wider debates by untangling social anxiety from its medicalised underpinnings, challenging and refashioning them in order to shape new perspectives for how academic and professional communities conceptualise and approach social anxiety and emotional distress more broadly. Crucially, it has centred the voices of those who live and navigate daily life with social anxiety. While not exhaustive, this book presents a thorough examination of the complex intersections between the spatialities, temporalities and embodiments of the anxious experience, conceptual threads which have been woven through the empirical heart of this book and are briefly summarised here.

Anxious spatialities

Social anxiety is a socially and spatially mediated phenomenon in which a person's sense of connectedness to and belongingness in a world shared with others is profoundly altered. First and foremost, drawing attention to the inherent spatialities re-centres the everyday social interactions, expectations and spaces that are fundamental not only to the early conceptualisations of social anxiety but lie at the very heart of its lived experience (Chapter 2). Examining the interactions between self, others and the myriad routines and environments that comprise daily life discloses a reciprocal and simultaneously *disrupted* and *disruptive* set of geographies that continuously shape ongoing and enduring experiences of anxious distress. Examining the situated aspects of social anxiety has drawn attention not only to the content and context of anxious distress but has enabled a deeper understanding of its complexity, one that is not limited to its restrictive and disruptive capacity, but is also attentive to the various ways it is enacted and sustained; its association with avoidance, withdrawal and isolation; feelings of uncertainty, disconnection and detachment; and the overwhelming social emptiness that often accompanies it. In addressing the experience of distress and its contexts, the stories embedded throughout this book have highlighted the diminishing and disruptive capacity of practices, encounters and spaces associated with everyday life that, for so many, confine and "chip away" at the self (Philo, 2017). It is evident that the social world is a source of intense fear in which everyday involvement is overwhelming, leading to a sense of embodied disruption that renders a person out of sync with and disconnected from the rhythms of social life. In order to avoid social threats, including disapproval, exclusion or rejection, many exist "on the fringes" (Scott, 2005), which often culminates in shrinking social and spatial worlds (Chapter 7). Yet, even as social worlds shrink and opportunities for social encounters diminish, anxiety persists.

Overall, social anxiety profoundly alters the coherent, habitual and embodied sense of being in and navigating through every day social and spatial worlds, but these aspects cannot be fully understood without addressing certain intrinsic temporalities bound into the condition.

Anxious temporalities

Social anxiety is constantly in motion as an embodied experience continuously marked by the revolutions of repetition and anticipation (Chapter 4). Examining the temporal aspects of social anxiety disrupts the notion that it occurs only as a succession of isolable events or occasional occurrences in a person's life, confined to the specific circumstances or conditions in which it arises with no broader or ongoing effects. The persistence and complexity of social anxiety are mirrored in its layered, restrictive and disruptive temporalities. It is this complexity that ensures anxiety's ungraspable, often unspeakable, motions. At the temporal core of the anxious experience are the indivisible entanglements of past, present and future, through which anxious distress is experienced and sustained.

Typically, anxiety leans *towards* the future as an excessive preoccupation with that which has not happened *yet*. Anticipation *throws* a person towards anxious expectations of a future that is hostile and threatening and acts to "presence" the innumerable *what ifs* that may lead to social rejection. The "future" also embodies an affective force that propels itself towards the "present" and through this imminence, the inevitability of the future, filled with "certain uncertainty", becomes inescapable. Anticipatory processes are typically associated with the capacity to *pre-empt, act on* and even *engineer* potential futures (Anderson, 2010). As discussed further below and outlined concretely in Chapter 8, people do indeed act upon them in myriad ways but the experiential dynamics of anticipation viewed here in the context of social anxiety as something that routinely disrupts and upends social life require further examination. While faced with the inevitability of the future, the force of social anxiety can also be felt in the persistence of the past-orientated movements of repetition and rumination. Memories of past experiences and adversities remain affectively rooted in the body, reigniting feelings of precarity that alert the individual to new or qualitatively similar social encounters. Such repetitions capture how the past comes back as a haunting by forcefully re-entering the present not as a fond memory but rather as a salient reminder of harsh social realities.

Deep-rooted memories also perceptively and affectively colour ruminations on "immediate past" interactions and events in which feelings of failure are so readily encountered. Ruminations narrow and re-affirm the social world as one of "outsidedness". This retrospectivity is typically only considered through its cognitive dimensions, as "thought ruminations" and not through its embodied insinuation into the "present" lifeworld of the individual. The embodied repetitions and enacted ruminations retroactively charges, even redraws, past events and adversities as traumatic (Chapter 4). Thus, the capacity to "sink into" the world is constantly uprooted, suspended between and constrained by the continuous impingement of the temporal movements of rumination and repetition on the one hand, and the anticipation of the future and its encroaching imminence, on the other. The present "presents" the individual with repeating scenarios of a humiliated and shamed self, one that is always faltering and failing at the point of human connection or simply being human. The minutiae of daily life provide infinite fodder for critical, self-reflexive ruminations for people with social anxiety. These temporalities are ultimately rooted in the embodiment of anxious distress.

Anxious embodiments

Social anxiety is a deeply embodied and affective phenomenon experienced, expressed and enacted in and through the body. By attending to the embodiments of anxious distress, these dimensions are resituated back into a narrative of experience and attended to as distressing and upsetting, yet inherently meaningful aspects, of people's anxious lives. These "intensities" – inclusive of the cognitive, the somatic and the behavioural dimensions of experience – often separated out and positioned as in need of "correction", coalesce to produce particular cycles of "embodied affectivity" (Fuchs and Koch, 2014, p. 508). Contributing to a small body of new research attending to experiential embodiments of distress (Vaughan *et al.*, 2022), the anxious body is reconceived here as a resonant body, one that is in many ways perhaps *too* attuned, *too* open to the infinite possibilities and affective qualities of the social world. As a consequence, the socially anxious person is propelled into self-protective action in order to limit or lessen the disorientating and debilitating impacts of the social world. The habitual practices of planning and other purposeful interventions (Chapter 8) can be viewed as creative negotiations with the intensities of social space, which are implemented to limit their negative impact and preserve some aspects of the self. This constant management and monitoring that sustains interaction in/with the social world can, however, be exhausting and deleterious. Social avoidance or, on the extreme end, social withdrawal are acts of resistance that force a deliberate "social change" and "slowing down" in the face of the multiple and multiplying embodied and temporal tensions (Chapter 4). Yet, despite the cyclical and persistent presence of social anxiety in a person's life, and the continuous negotiations undertaken, these practices are never seamlessly habituated into the routines of daily life, and rather they continue – as habitually revisited, reappraised and consequential for routine decision-making – to rupture the fabric of everyday life and spaces.

Avenues for future research

The findings of this book not only answer questions about living with social anxiety, they also prompt new lines of questioning. Some suggestions for future areas of research are outlined here.

The consequences of social anxiety over the life course, or at certain stages of a person's life, emerges in various ways throughout the qualitative materials herein, including in the barriers faced to help-seeking (Chapter 5), in the consequences for employment opportunities (Chapter 7) and in the steady shrinking of people's social and spatial worlds (Chapters 6 and 7). While evident in the data, the longer-term machinations of social anxiety were not a specific focus of this research. Qualitative approaches to the life course can help to uncover the critical periods and cumulative personal, social and environmental circumstances, which, over time, enable social anxiety to flourish (Pearce, 2018). Embracing both past episodes and future trajectories can offer unique insights into how social anxiety is aligned with particular social patterns, values and norms. By extension, such an approach could examine how anxious individuals "by their socialisation, adapt[...] to the structures of the social worlds that they inhabit" and the varied ways this is suffused with specifically anxious "biographical trajectories" (Malmberg and Andersson, 2023, p. 463).

Another broader thread relates to the evident and remarkable sense of disconnection and loss communicated throughout the stories shared with this research. Everyday worlds are infused with social comparisons of "not being good enough" and a feeling of "out-of-placeness". Social worlds are often marked by a profound sense of emptiness and opportunities for connection, as well as future ambitions, hopes and dreams are closed off. Yet, there is a sense of yearning for the unpursued, lost or never-gained aspects of social life. Fruitful avenues of further research, taking cue from recent "negative" geographies (Bissell, Rose and Harrison, 2021), could illuminate these aspects of life that are "unlived", missed, invisible and *non*-emergent.

Recommendations for policy and practice

> What greater scourge could befall psychiatry than becoming imper-
> sonal – which means losing sight of the persona of the patient? The
> great technological advances that have taken place in medicine within
> the last three-quarter century raise this threat – the loss of the per-
> sonal relationship with the patient. The whole tradition is based on
> healing and caring for the sick as persons, through constant personal
> contact between the doctor and the patient.
>
> (Bartemeier, 1952, p. 1 *cited in* Pickersgill, 2019, p. 19)

First and foremost, this book stresses the importance of understanding the personal geographies of those living with social anxiety. With this in mind, there are
two interrelated recommendations for policy and practice with the goal of reclaim-
ing, what Bartemeier contends, has been lost. These recommendations involve
giving due consideration to experiential knowledge and re-centring therapeutic
and collaborative relationships within mental healthcare settings and beyond.

This research bears witness to the capabilities people with social anxiety
have for understanding and communicating what is going on in their personal
and emotional lives and capturing in detail the aggravating conditions and
contexts of their social and spatial worlds. In light of this, the findings of this
research explicitly caution against the most recent guidance outlined in the
DSM-V (2013) (Chapter 2) that shifts decision-making power further into the
hands of the clinician and risks dismissing, or even denying, the subjectivity
and agency of the socially anxious person. Alternative approaches to diagnosis
such as "formulations" should also be considered (Johnstone and Dallos,
2013), where people are engaged in "a process of ongoing and collaborative
sense-making" (Harper and Moss, 2003, p. 4) with a mental health professional. In addition to this, help-seeking is recognised as a long and often arduous process for a socially anxious person who must navigate numerous barriers
to care and support (Chapter 5). Given the length of time taken to seek support, social fears are deep-rooted in habitual patterns of distress. Current mental health promotion campaigns and interventions across the UK, shaped by
neoliberal imperatives of responsibility and self-reliance (Teghtsoonian, 2009),
present severe limitations in that they are typically short-term, and becoming
increasingly self-directed delivered through online cognitive behavioural therapy courses. Short-term therapies do not provide sufficient time for the socially
anxious to build rapport or trust with a designated therapist. Self-directed
therapies are near-void of interpersonal contact with a therapist, who provides
crucial sources of guidance, compassion and support. With these issues in
mind, an emphasis must be placed on reducing the barriers to care and promoting patient-centred care to ensure the content and contexts of people's
anxious experiences are acknowledged and addressed. Furthermore, the development of longer-term therapeutic relationships and interpersonal connections should be promoted to ensure people feel adequately supported.

As will be highlighted in the next section, the kind of "therapeutic work" afforded by attention to and representation of anxious distress should not be considered ancillary to treatment and/or recovery, but rather serve as a central strategy to understanding how social and spatial life is lived, endured and managed at various times and in various places by people living with social anxiety. Therapeutic approaches should acknowledge the often diminished and difficult social worlds of those living with social anxiety. As this book has outlined, there is a tendency of people to internalise and ruminate over negative social interactions as well as to criticise and socially isolate themselves. Finding creative ways for mental health experiences to be "externalised" and "made object", for example, through written word, can be an effective way of reconvening and then processing with distress and emotional suffering (Rian and Hammer, 2013, p. 678). In addition to this, and in recognition of the embodiments of distress outlined above, the promotion of therapeutic interventions that deeply and viscerally contradict the feelings of isolation, loneliness and alienation could also help to foster more "positive" embodiments and relationships with the self and others. Similar movement-based practices and (psycho)therapies have been explored, for example, yoga for anorexia nervosa (Lucas, 2022) as an integrative approach for those experiencing distressing bodily disconnections. Finally, the diminished social worlds of people with social anxiety (Chapter 7) are often disconnected from the communal rhythms and synchronicity of civic and daily life and marked by feelings of isolation and loneliness. Social prescribing initiatives could help to foster civic engagement and active community involvement. Connecting people with their local communities could encourage individuals to become more integrated into those communities, fostering a sense of belonging and reducing social isolation (Bell *et al.*, 2019). This connection could encourage new ways of inhabiting existing spaces that enable people to break from the anxious time loops of recall, anticipation and avoidance and foster more positive instances of social connection and interaction. The provision of safe spaces may enable people to disclose and challenge isolating and oppressive personal and social conditions that exacerbate their experiences of distress and offer crucial alternatives to medicalising them (Doblytė, 2022). With all the recommendations outlined here, it is absolutely critical to provide dedicated support and guidance as people engage in therapeutic and/or social interventions. By doing so, we can ensure that they do not continue to navigate the challenges of social anxiety alone and instead find the necessary support, empowerment and community to live well *with* social anxiety.

Unsung impacts

It is important to consider the small-scale impacts of this the research on those who participated in it. Research participants were incredibly supportive of, and enthusiastic about, a research project that was solely about their, largely neglected, lived experiences, one that worked with their anxieties both practically, in terms of non-face-to-face methods, and conceptually, by viewing social anxiety through a more personal lens. The opportunity to discuss experiences of mental and emotional distress – and to have someone listen attentively with genuine care and interest – may be empowering and cathartic, enabling a sense of ownership over experiences that are so often dismissed, ignored or marginalised. In addition to being "listened to", participants are also motivated by the prospect that sharing their experiences will help others living with social anxiety, and their family members, friends and colleagues understand the often uncertain and distressing aspects of social life. At the end of the questionnaires and during the interviews, participants often told me that they had enjoyed participating in the research, and indeed were grateful that someone was interested in, listening to and working with their "voices" of experience:

> [The questionnaire] made me ask myself a lot of questions I wouldn't normally ask myself because of my lack of positive self-dialogue.
>
> (Jane, QR)

> I appreciate the questionnaire's inclusion of anecdotal information. It has been useful to reflect. It has helped me to identify what is a problem that I had identified before as belonging to other areas of my life, so thank you.
>
> (Hannah, QR)

> It's been really nice talking to you knowing you understand and aren't judging me. Thank you for doing this work. It's so important!
>
> (Lucy, IR)

> It's been really helpful for me. It's actually given me a fresh perspective on my anxiety, I'm going to take a copy of this interview to my therapist next week and talk it through with her.
>
> (Jo, IR)

These impacts may indeed seem small but, for me, they are the most significant in highlighting the importance of this research. If not for participant's willingness to discuss the often difficult-to-articulate, deeply personal and emotional aspects of their mental health, my efforts to humanise and capture the intensity and uncertainty of socially anxious worlds would not have been possible. I hope in some small way that this book does justice to the stories so readily shared with this research and brings to light a little-known social geography of social anxiety, a geography otherwise anxiously hidden to the detriment of many.

References

American Psychiatric Association (2013) *Diagnostic and Statistical Manual of Mental Disorders*. 5th Edition. Washington, DC: American Psychiatric Association. https://doi.org/10.1176/appi.books.9780890425596

Anderson, B. (2010) 'Preemption, precaution, preparedness: Anticipatory action and future geographies', *Progress in Human Geography*, 34(6), pp. 777–798. https://doi.org/10.1177/0309132510362600

Bell, S.L. et al. (2019) 'The "healthy dose" of nature: A cautionary tale', *Geography Compass*, 13(1), p. e12415. https://doi.org/10.1111/gec3.12415

Bissell, D., Rose, M. and Harrison, P. (eds) (2021) *Negative Geographies: Exploring the Politics of Limits*. Lincol: University of Nebraska Press.

Deacon, B.J. (2013) 'The biomedical model of mental disorder: A critical analysis of its validity, utility, and effects on psychotherapy research', *Clinical Psychology Review*, 33(7), pp. 846–861. https://doi.org/10.1016/j.cpr.2012.09.007

Deacon, B.J. and McKay, D. (2015) 'The biomedical model of psychological problems: A call for critical dialogue', *The Behavior Therapist*, 38(7), pp. 231–235.

Doblytė, S. (2022) '"The almighty pill and the blessed healthcare provider": Medicalisation of mental distress from an Eliasian perspective', *Social Theory & Health*, 20(4), pp. 363–379. https://doi.org/10.1057/s41285-021-00165-1

Fitzgerald, D. and Callard, F. (2015) 'Social science and neuroscience beyond interdisciplinarity: Experimental entanglements', *Theory, Culture & Society*, 32(1), pp. 3–32. https://doi.org/10.1177/0263276414537319

Fuchs, T. and Koch, S.C. (2014) 'Embodied affectivity: On moving and being moved', *Frontiers in Psychology*, 5, p. 508. https://doi.org/10.3389/fpsyg.2014.00508

Harper, D. and Moss, D. (2003) 'A different kind of chemistry? Reformulating "formulation"', pp. 6–10.

Johnstone, L. and Dallos, R. (2013) *Formulation in Psychology and Psychotherapy: Making Sense of People's Problems*. London: Taylor & Francis Group. http://ebookcentral. proquest.com/lib/gla/detail.action?docID=1319025 (Accessed: 17 October 2023).

Liebowitz, M.R. et al. (1985) 'Social phobia. Review of a neglected anxiety disorder', *Archives of General Psychiatry*, 42(7), pp. 729–736. https://doi.org/10.1001/archpsyc.1985.01790300097013

Lucas, G. (2022) 'Moving matters: Living in the body after anorexia', in H. Lewis et al. (eds) *The Practical Handbook of Eating Difficulties: A Comprehensive Guide from Personal and Professional Perspectives*. Shoreham-by-Sea: Pavilion, pp. 331–338.

Malmberg, B. and Andersson, E.K. (2023) 'Exploring life-course Trajectories in local spatial contexts across Sweden', *Annals of the American Association of Geographers*, 113(2), pp. 448–468. https://doi.org/10.1080/24694452.2022.2105684

Pearce, J.R. (2018) 'Complexity and uncertainty in geography of health research: Incorporating life-course perspectives', *Annals of the American Association of Geographers*, 108(6), pp. 1491–1498. https://doi.org/10.1080/24694452.2017.1416280

Philo, C. (2017) Less-than-human geographies. *Political Geography*, 60, pp. 256–258. https://doi.org/10.1016/j.polgeo.2016.11.014

Pickersgill, M. (2019) 'Digitising psychiatry? Sociotechnical expectations, performative nominalism and biomedical virtue in (digital) psychiatric praxis', *Sociology of Health & Illness*, 41(S1), pp. 16–30. https://doi.org/10.1111/1467-9566.12811

Rian, J. and Hammer, R. (2013) The practical application of narrative medicine at Mayo Clinic: Imagining the scaffold of a worthy house. *Culture, Medicine, and Psychiatry*, 37(4), pp. 670–680.

Rose, N. (2006) 'Disorders without borders? The expanding scope of psychiatric practice', *Biosocieties*, 1, pp. 465–484. https://doi.org/10.1017/S1745855206004078

Scott, S. (2005) 'The red, shaking fool: Dramaturgical dilemmas in shyness', *Symbolic Interaction*, 28(1), pp. 91–110. https://doi.org/10.1525/si.2005.28.1.91

Teghtsoonian, K. (2009) 'Depression and mental health in neoliberal times: A critical analysis of policy and discourse', *Social Science & Medicine (1982)*, 69(1), pp. 28–35. https://doi.org/10.1016/j.socscimed.2009.03.037

Vaughan, P. et al. (2022) '"Chains weigh heavy": Body mapping embodied experiences of anxiety', *The Qualitative Report* [Preprint]. https://doi.org/10.46743/2160-3715/2023.5712

Index

For Product Safety Concerns and Information please contact our EU
representative GPSR@taylorandfrancis.com
Taylor & Francis Verlag GmbH, Kaufingerstraße 24, 80331 München, Germany